EVERY DAY YOGA

Ten Minutes a Day
to Keep the Doctor Away

It is my dream to share my love, respect, and joy for this ancient healing practice with the world. It is my hope that this exchange will help to transform the world by empowering individuals physically, mentally, and spiritually.

Callico Publishing

callicopublishing@gmail.com

Contents

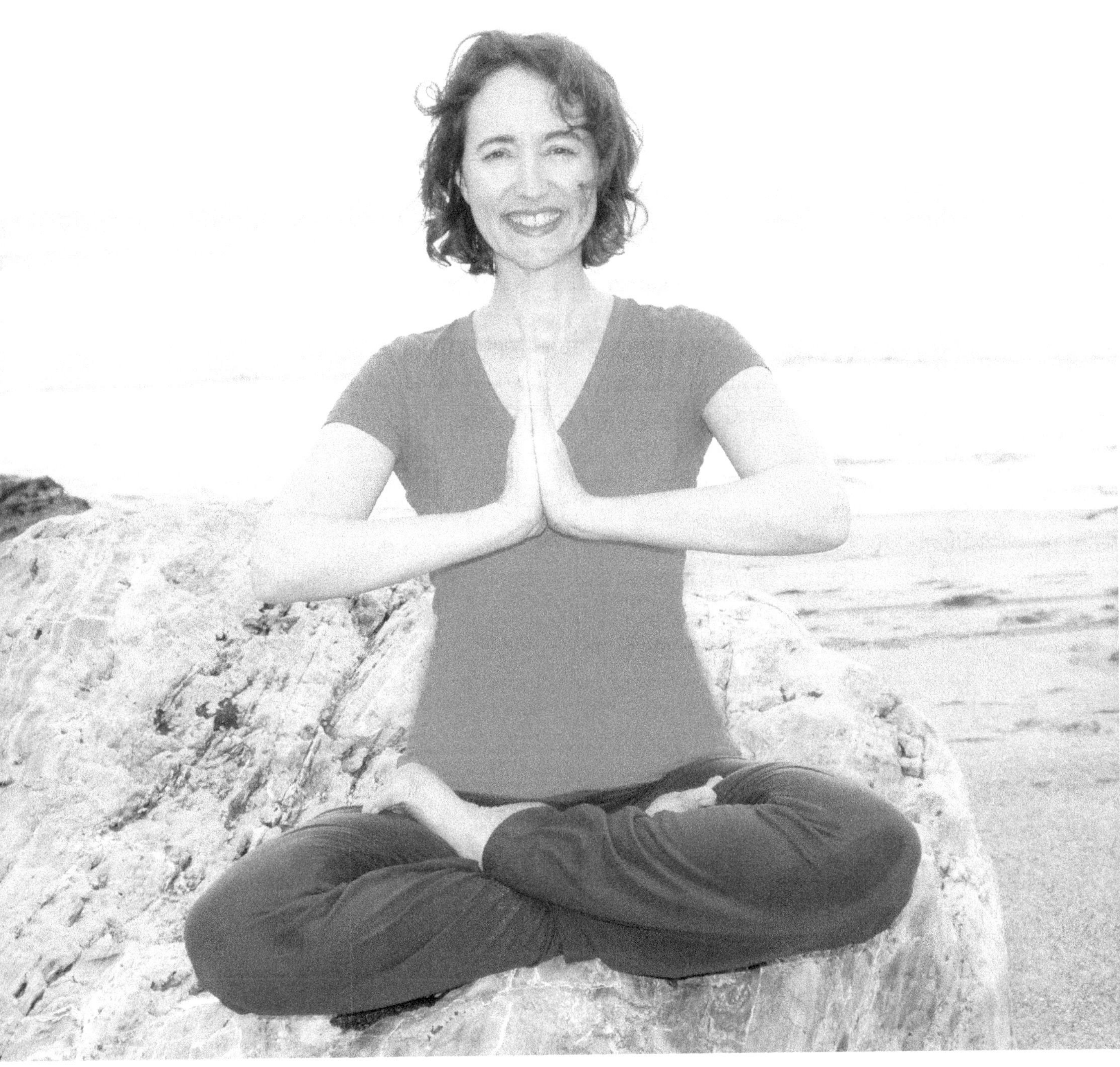

Sitting in Lotus Pose, *Padmasana*

Kritajna, the sanskrit word for gratitude is made up of two words. *Krita* meaning cultivated, and *jna* which is a state of consciousness.

Kritajna is about cultivating awareness of consciousness so we can be fully present to enjoy the gift of each precious moment.

Gratitude

I would like to thank all the yoga teachers and gurus who have and are still propagating the philosophies and proven techniques of yoga for the enhancement and betterment of society. One of those was a pioneer yoga teacher in New Orleans, Alvina Haverkamp, who took great care in making sure I performed postures correctly. I'd also like to thank Patanjali for compiling the Yoga Sutras; Yogi Bhajan and Gurumukh for being a light in the yoga world of Kundalini; Pattabhi Jois for his vigorous Ashtanga school of yoga; and B.K.S.Iyengar for sharing his vast knowledge of yoga in his many books and for his enlightened words on expanding the practice.

I'd like to thank my friends; Allan Ferro for his encouragement and for educating me on Photoshop, In-Design, cover editing, and patience through this process; Merilly Ruglas for working on the first versions of cover layout, which kept me encouraged; Richard Wegmen for sharing many sessions of yoga and meditation with me and for always being a jovial soul; Owen Romero for believing in me even when I couldn't believe in myself; and Larry LaFluer for his beautiful depiction of me in meditation on this cover and his friendship.

I would also like to sincerely thank Dragan Bilic for the beautiful layout of this book and for his patience with me in waiting for pages this past year; Lorraine Eberts for her careful reading and suggestions for transforming content; Mia Lett for encouragement, notes and for allowing her sweet daughters to take care of Molly Dolly while I travel promoting this book; Julie Loper for her detailed editing and suggestions; and Annie Sergi and Jen Ramos for generously posing for the photos for this book.

Lastly, I'd like to thank my Buddhist community, the SGI, Soka Gaika International, and the members specifically in Venice, Sherman Oaks, California and New Orleans, Louisiana for their uplifting life examples and encouragement; my friend and fellow Buddhist Val erie Sauchelli for being a living example of infinite possibilities and positivity no matter what her health or external circumstances might have appeared; Amelia Stone for sharing phone calls and observations about life; and Daisuka Ikeda for being a living example of the "winning spirit" and his determination to help others succeed and live joyfully to ultimately transform the world with the lotus flowers of compassion and peace.

There are so many others I'd like to thank for the conception, inspiration and encouragement of this book. If you have met me in life, I am thanking you here. Your kind words and peaceful remarks have made it to this page. I am grateful for all who have shared this existence with me.

Dedication

This book is dedicated to the recently deceased Dasaku Ikeda and to some of my dear friends and family who were caught in the web between life and death and have peacefully surrendered to continuing this journey on the other side of the river. The caricature of me doing yoga on the front cover was created by my friend Larry LaFluer, who passed away of cancer in January of 2013. He was neither aware of the dangers of the common fast food American diet nor aware of the fatal consequences of extreme stress and how the negative influences of others can harm the body, mind, and soul. He is one of the reasons I wish for the world to have the knowledge and the tools for peaceful, healthy living. We all must leave this earth at some point in our lives; but living with courage and strength and health and vitality should be our birthright. And with a few adjustments, peace and happiness can at least be on everyone's horizon. Peace is a treasure, and the only place to find it is within.

It was discovered later in his life that my father was born with a defective heart valve. He had his first heart attack at seventeen, experimental bypass surgery at thirty-three, and passed away at the young age of forty-seven. He is dear to my heart and a catalyst for writing this book. He tried many different diets and methods, but ultimately living a stagnant life, overweight and slowly dying, finally caught up to him. His seesaw ride on and off smoking cigarettes took its toll on his body and spirit as well. A few years before he passed away, the one thing he tried that seemed to work was the Pritikin diet, which consisted mostly of salads and vegetables. One more piece of wellbeing that must have helped him was walking our beloved dog, Tannin, every day. He lost weight and was thinner than he had been in his adult life. But change is not easy. For some change may seem like an omen. I saw a shade of sadness in his eyes that I hadn't seen before. A few weeks later, he gave up on his diet and went back to his old familiar habits. Within a few months he was back to his previous weight with a few added pounds and stresses. Many years later, I realized that living in this way, sick, tired, and overweight was all he had known for so many years. Losing weight and having more energy may have been completely out of his comfort zone. The most difficult challenges we will face in life are the ones that come from within.

Notes of Caution

This book is not meant to usurp any medical treatment you are receiving nor is it designed to give you any medical advice. On the contrary, it is designed to empower you to be the best you can be and to enhance your physical, mental, and spiritual wellbeing. It is recommended that if you are receiving treatment for injuries, you should consult your chiropractor or doctor about any constraints to your practice.

If you are seeing a doctor, you have even more reason to begin practicing yoga. Human life can be enhanced by a minimal practice of yoga and by living yogic philosophies. For example, consider the entire human race living the philosophy of Ahimsa, the principle of non-violence, for themselves and others. Eating proper nutrition and moving the body to heal and relieve stress is a form of practicing non-violence. Perhaps all life on our planet might benefit from a healthy, happy, holy human race.

Moving the body in new and improved ways releases stuck energy that lies dormant in the muscles, creating resistance to practice, and may expose hidden emotions. "Yoga tears," as some yogis call this experience, are normal. With daily practice and heartfelt communication, we can work through these issues to heal, not only mentally, but any physical manifestations of these hidden resentments and emotions. Louis Hay's break-through book, *You Can Heal Your Life*, outlines the connections between emotions and their physical manifestations. Blocked emotions often result in disease. In Hay's book, she writes about her own experience with cancer and eventual recovery, a recovery that she says could not have happened without realizing the connection between the emotional baggage she carried around and the effect of this baggage on her body. Practicing yoga is a powerful way to release and heal old injuries and old resentments so that we can clear a path for a healthy future.

Along the way, perhaps discovering our true selves is our mission. This journey may not be easy, and for some, it may even seem treacherous. But it is beautiful, I assure you.

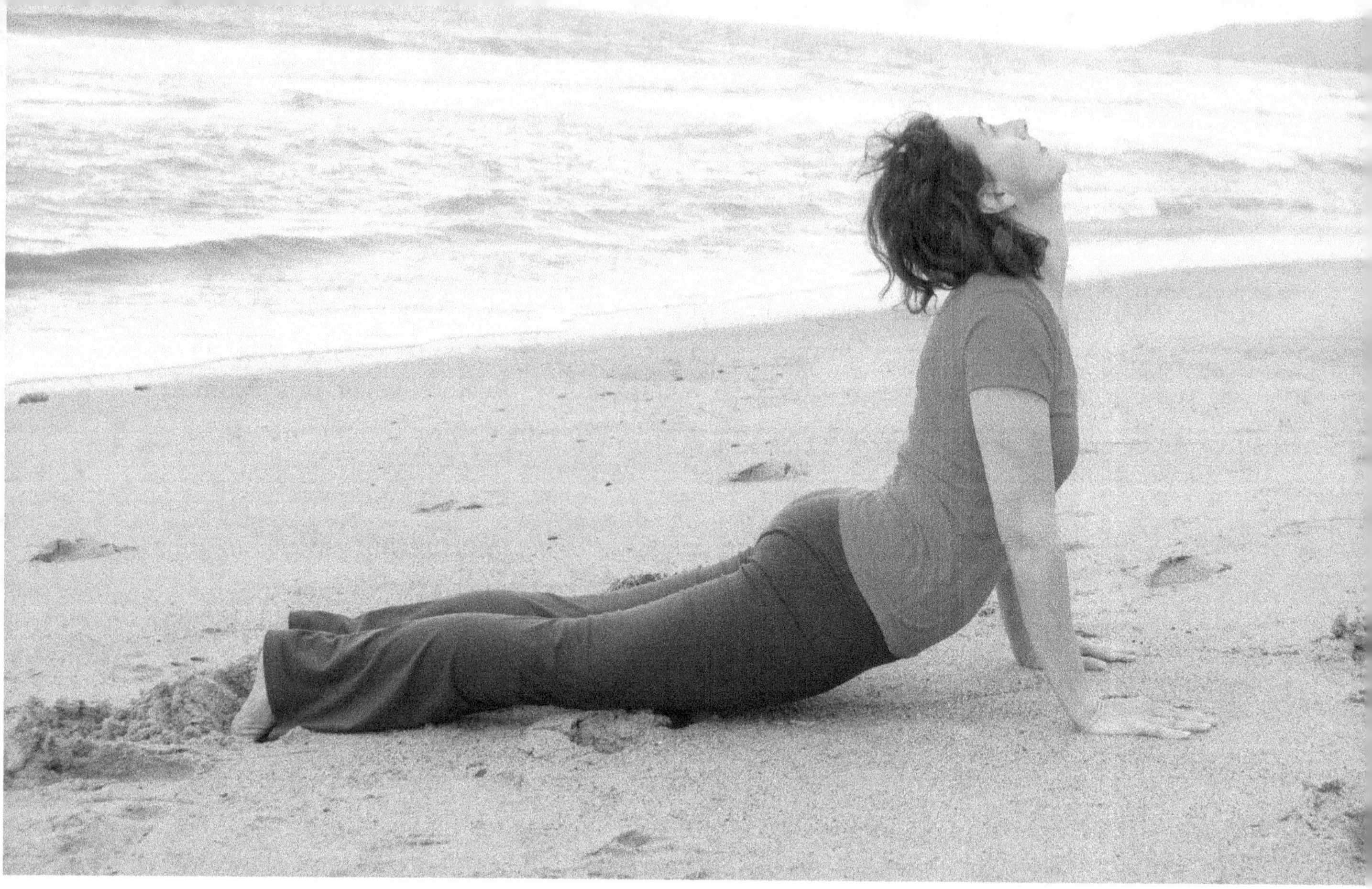

Stretching in Up-Dog Pose, *Urdhva Mukha Svanasana*

Beginnings are often the most challenging part of progress and transformation. Once the train is in motion, it is much easier to maintain. Once it stops, it must work up the initial energy to begin again and again and again.

Momentum creates more energy, so taking time throughout our day to move the body and calm the, for many, overactive brain muscle may help us overcome obstacles and make wise decisions. Stagnant energy creates an unhealthy environment. Yoga movement and philosophy are ways to maintain a happy, healthy, holy energy.

An Intro to the Book

I began writing this book in 2008 to process my own practice and as a response to my own resistance to my normal hour and a half daily yoga practice. After a series of personal and professional challenges and the fallout that often occurs in the process, I realized what I was missing in my life. My daily practice had slipped to once or twice a week.

For the newcomers to yoga, remember that beginning anything new comes with challenges. When learning to play guitar my fingers had to build up little calluses, which was a painful process. However, after just one month of lessons, beautiful sounds began to emerge out of my guitar. This great pleasure could not have been experienced without the pain of developing calluses and the frustration of learning something new.

I often encounter people who tell me they just don't have time for yoga or meditation. I may ask them, "So you have time to drive in traffic, work for your boss all day, support your friend by hearing his band in the evening, but you don't have ten minutes a day for yourself?" I soon realized that within this seemingly insignificant measure of time could be the seeds of something great: sanity, peace of mind, and finding truth in a muddled world. And just like the price of this book compared with all the money wasted on useless endeavors, ten minutes a day is a small price to pay for the benefits of a lifetime of practice.

When the body is not accustomed to certain movements, people often resist the pain that may occur from this new activity. This is one reason for beginning your yoga practice with ten minutes a day, which is enough time to receive significant benefits, but not enough time to cause harm or burn-out. Still, even ten minutes of new movements may result in some muscle pains. These pains will thankfully not compare to going to the gym for three hours, once a week, only to suffer the effects of this strain for the rest of the week.

When people plunge into new activities with too much vigor, they are often deflated before their bodies have a chance to adjust or to receive the benefits of the new activity. Starting small and building a daily practice will yield far more results than any intense sporadic exercise program. However, with yoga, you do not have to build more than ten-minutes a day to receive lifelong benefits and to expand in your practice.

In yoga, "no pain, no gain," is not a precept. You are not expected to push yourself beyond your limits to receive, in some cases, immediate benefits. Once, I tried a new coach at a gym and told him that I had previously had bad experiences with coaches because they would ask me to do so many squats or quadricep exercises that I would be very sore for days and often the rest of the week. In our session he specifically focused on these types of exercise. I did not feel pain in the moment, but in the next few days my legs felt bruised, and I could barely walk. I felt as if someone had beaten my muscles with a bat. I did not go to that coach again. This idea that causing pain is somehow productive is counterintuitive to living happy, healthy, and holy. Compassion begins with ourselves.

In Yoga, you are expected to be present with where you are at this moment and to have compassion for a body that does so much for you; words cannot accurately express the wonder of the billions of biological adjustments and communications happening right now in each human body. Students often express experiencing immediate benefits from their yoga practice, which come in the form of feeling lighter, happier, stronger, and more centered.

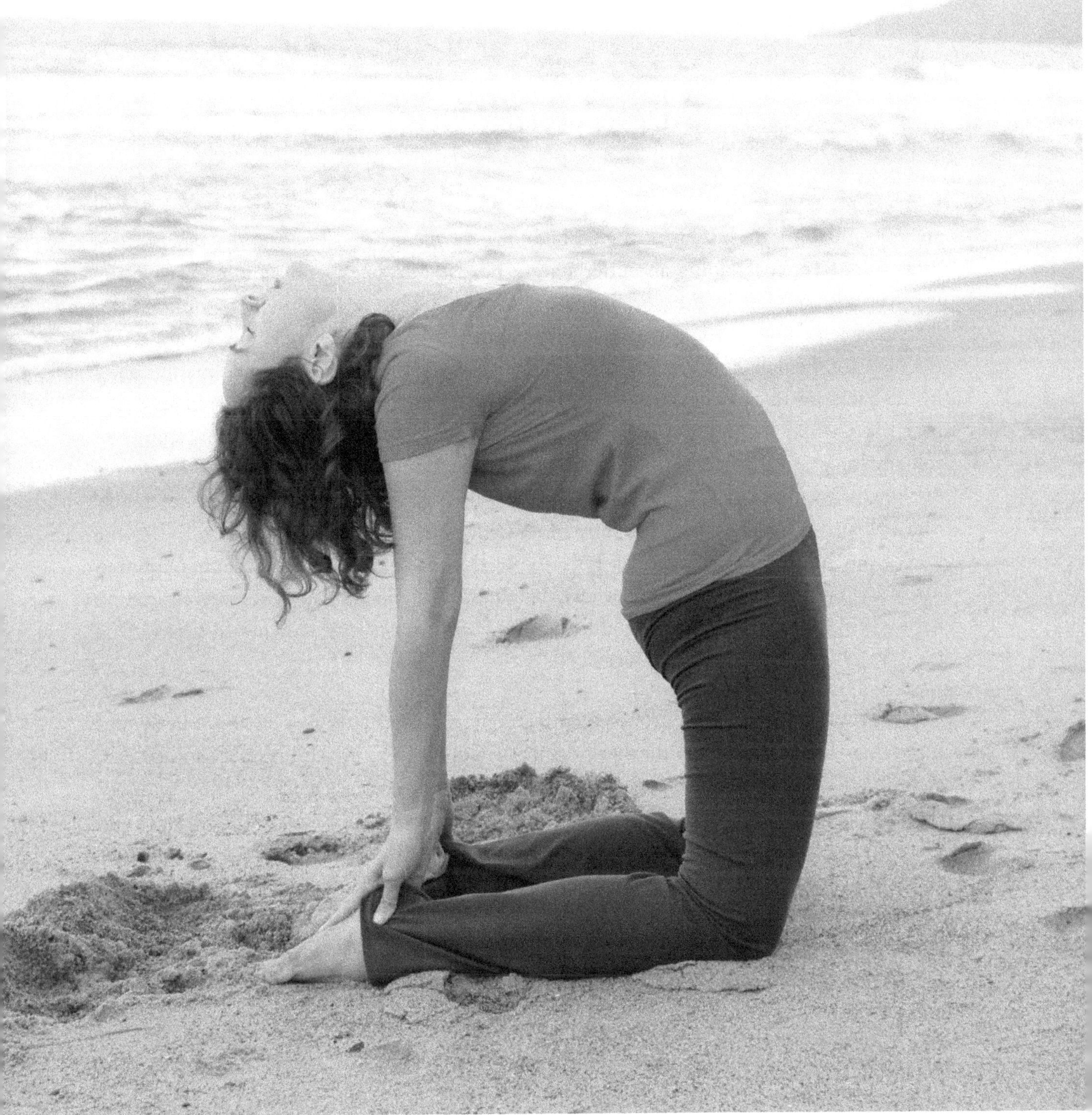

Expanding the heart in Camel Pose, *Ustrasana*

So many people are wrapped in the warm, cozy, and sometimes even thorny blanket of who they think they are. What if our identities were expanded in the service of others?

About the Author

In reviewing my own history of yoga, I had to acknowledge that I began my yoga practice as a child, frequently doing shoulder stands, headstands, backbends, and even covering my eyes with my feet in *Raja Bhujangasana* or King Cobra pose while lying on the floor watching television. I would perform back bends pretending to be a crab walking across the floor for the delight of my younger siblings. It was not uncommon to find me tumbling in the backyard in cartwheels and walkovers. Finally, my mother enlisted me in an acrobatic class, where she thought I could learn more. I was later injured because my spine had folded almost in half attempting an acrobatic contortion. Unlike acrobats or other forms of circus acts or performances, when practicing yoga, you do not have to be a contortionist. The ancient yogis believe yoga is a form of natural, creative movement of the body. It is the body's way of healing and expressing itself. For this reason, we can observe that children often do yoga naturally. After my sister's daughter, Danielle, was born, she was stretching her body in the incubator into a modified, *Adho Mukha Svanasana*, Downward Facing Dog pose. Yes, I was astonished.

One of the most amazing parts of a yoga practice is meditation or sitting quietly and observing the breath. To my mother's dismay, I had an uncanny ability to disappear into states of calm, simply by noticing a falling leaf or looking up at the sky at the wonder of the metamorphosing shapes of the clouds. Children are full of wonder at the simple and seemingly ordinary small moments in life. Perhaps after years of programing and forgetting this beautiful infinite state, we need a practice to help us remember what we've always known, that we are connected to all that is and all that was and all that will be. My mother would insist that I come back to earth, as she put it. I did not realize until years later, that those moments of peace were moments of meditation and what adults were looking for in quiet time.

Around thirty years ago, I began the journey of returning to that joyful, inspired, place young children often find so natural, my "true self" or *Satnam*. I was recovering from an accident when my friend's mother, Martha, purchased eight lessons of yoga for me for my birthday. The teacher, Alvina Haverkamp, a former ballet dancer, was precise and nurturing in her teaching, ensuring that I used modified poses to protect my neck from further injuries. I began to gain back some of the mobility and strength that I had prior to my accident. From that point, I purchased tapes and began learning not only yoga, but also Qigong and other healing and energy practices. Later, I participated in Melanie Fawer's Ashtanga workshop and practiced this form of yoga for several years. A friend asked me what I was doing to look so amazing. I said, "Yoga." She had no idea that yoga could do "all that."

In 2000, my enthusiasm and joy for my own practice blossomed into a desire to teach others. That year I became a certified yoga teacher. My first teaching assignment was to assist a Kundalini teacher who was seven months pregnant. She taught the class while I demonstrated the poses. I began reading and learning more about Kundalini Yoga. For several years Kundalini Yoga became my daily practice. I am certain that through these precious moments on the mat, I found not only myself again, but a more peaceful world.

On the morning of 9-11, after my yoga practice, I opened a book by Jon Kabat-Zen entitled *Wherever You Go, There You Are*. I wrote in my meditation journal (before I knew about the attacks) "Ahimsa, easy on your friends, but what about your enemies." Before I heard the war mongering political propaganda, I felt that the United States was on the precipice of great transformation for ourselves and the rest of the planet. I envisioned our country making choices that would reveal its true great character to the world. However, I was disappointed in the aftermath of all the knee jerk, mindless and spiritually void political decisions that followed. Because of my yoga practice, my perceptions of violence, both from the inside and from external sources were forever changed. I knew that violence was an inside job. I became even more driven to illuminate healthy, peaceful, and joyful individuals. In Buddhism, there is a philosophical saying that our external environment is merely a mirror image of our internal environment. The macrocosm reflects the microcosm, another reason for the importance of infusing the healing aspects of a daily yoga practice into the lives of all human beings.

Life without my yoga practice would have been very different and less inspired. Yoga has helped to keep me centered especially through the events like divorces, job changes, and catastrophic events like Hurricane Katrina. I acknowledge this mind, body, and soul practice for taking me through the rough stuff of life, whole, intact, and able to love.

Speaking of soul, yoga is a non-denominational, physical, mental, and spiritual practice, another feature that led me on to this path. I often practice Hindu mantras, repeated seed sounds and ancient words, in my meditation. I've also practiced the Buddhist mantras described in week six and one of my favorites from a Kundalini practice that I describe in week three of this book. I have also read and meditated on the words of Christian and Hebrew mystics. Yoga philosophies transcend religion without stepping on anyone's toes.

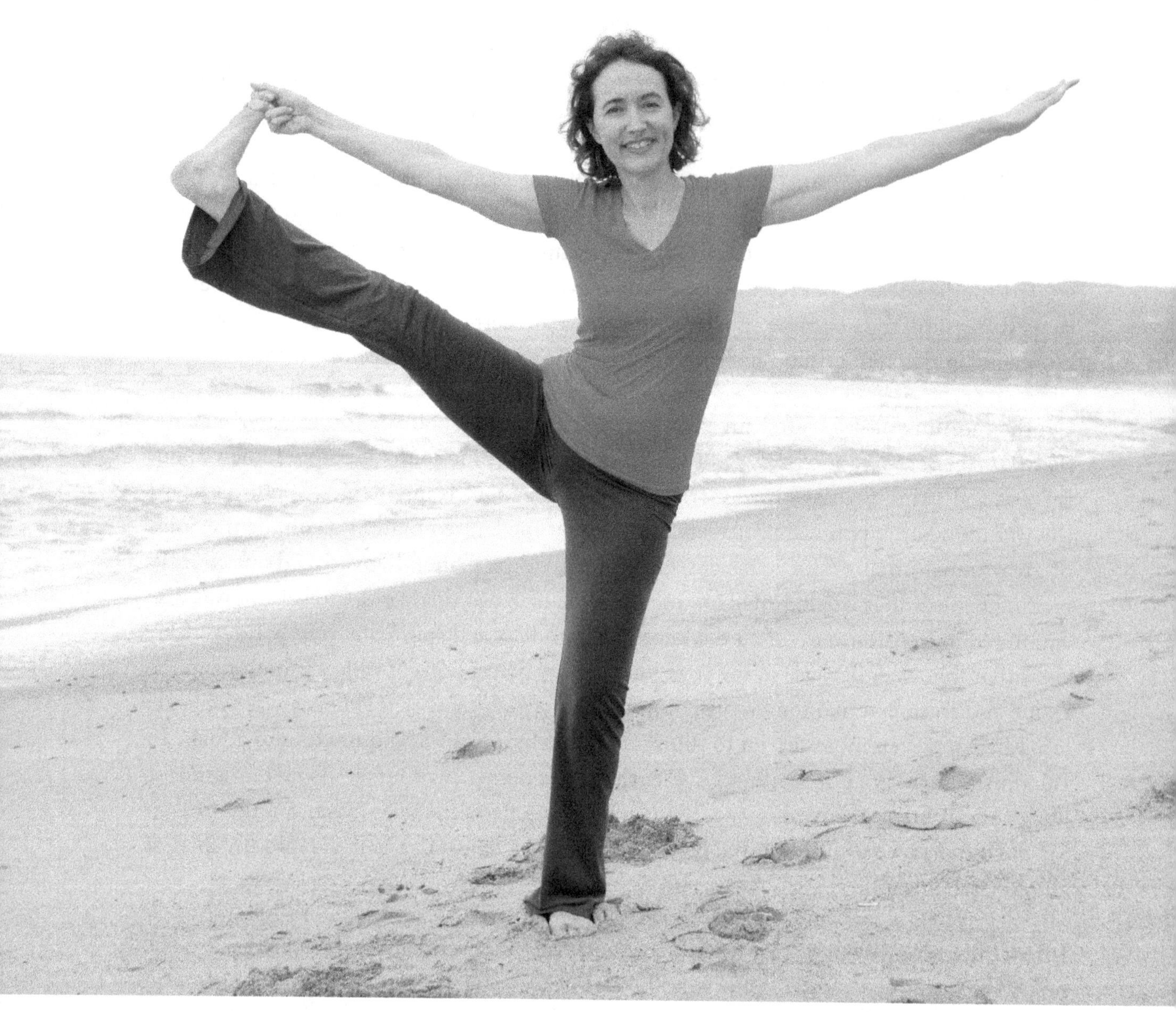

Reaching in Hand-to-Big-Toe Pose, *Utthita Hasta Padangusthasana*

Yoga is to Yoke together all the different elements of existence into one. It's an ancient holistic practice for mind, body, and soul that everyone, including those with religious or non-religious ideologies can enjoy.

What Is Yoga?

Yoga is many things to many people. Its roots are thousands of years old, stemming from the heart of India. This book is not designed to give you a history or theory of yoga. There are many books on this subject; some of the best are listed in "A Few Favorites." Yoga theory is far too extensive a subject for these few pages to encompass.

However, no explanation of yoga would be complete without mentioning *The Yoga Sutras of Patanjali*, which contain the *Eight Limbs of Yoga*, and are some of the earliest known texts on yoga. These eight limbs, or the eight-fold path, are the foundation of the philosophies of yoga. The first limb is *Yama*, regarding moral behavior towards others. The second is *Niyama*, regarding moral behavior towards oneself. The third is *Asana*, the physical practice of yoga postures. The fourth is *Pranayama*, breathing exercises. The fifth limb is *Pratyahara*, the withdrawal of the senses from the external world, so that the external is not a distraction to the internal. These are the seeds of modern meditation. What naturally follows meditation is the sixth limb, *Dharana*, which expounds concentration and the ability to focus on something uninterrupted by internal or external forces. Next is *Dhyana*, which is all-encompassing meditation. If *Dharana* is to focus on a single point, *Dyhana* is to focus on the universal, the omnipotent and eternal. These two are likened to the microcosm and the macrocosm, which in Buddhism and yoga are one in the same. The last limb is *Samadhi*, or bliss, the oneness of the self with the universe, also known in Buddhism as enlightenment.

Since Patanjali's time, yoga has grown and been expounded by many different teachers and philosophers. Still the roots of the eight-fold path are evident in all forms of yoga. The disciplines and physical practices are what make up most of the variations of teachings. Yoga styles are like cooking styles, mixed with sprinkles of various yoga ideologies with a smidgen of the individual's spice of life. Yoga is not only an experience we have on a mat; it is a way of life. For this reason, I am including recipes at the end this book to assist practitioners in healing and living a balanced, healthy lifestyle.

The practice of yoga has remained for thousands of years a way of life that is beneficial to the individual's physical, mental, and spiritual wellbeing and therefore the wellbeing of the world. Even though yoga is non-denominational, there are many Sanskrit mantras that can be incorporated into your practice. For those who prefer a more robust flavor to their practice, these mantras can be the added spice.

Yoga, as mentioned earlier, is also non-violent. Rather than creating a war with the body, as in many forms of exercise, a war that we can never win, we are asked to find peace from within. Yoga practitioners are not asked to overextend themselves to prove that they are somebody. You already are somebody.

The philosophy of yoga is to bring you closer to the person you already are, your true self or *Satnam*, pronounced like "but mom." You are not asked to become anything other than what you already are. You are asked to be with the person you are, feeling the breath and muscles and listening to your thoughts as an observer. You are the wise, compassionate, loving, mystical observer. That is you. "I am that I am."

The goal is to breathe into each pose and to be present with the breath and the body for a few precious moments. As your body becomes more familiar with the practice, how you perceive yourself practicing poses will change, freeing you to go deeper into poses and into your practice. By being present, you are creating more precious aware moments in your life. When I say aware, I am referring to being awake.

It is a common practice in our current society to go from one thought, idea, job, or advertisement to the next, without ever giving any of them much thought. This unawareness can lead to unwanted material input into the programs of our minds. Being unaware can wreak havoc on our potential in life. We may spend too much time on a train of thought, a train that we hold onto so tightly that we miss our next stop. Being unable to pull ourselves away from the mayhem of our minds, we may forget to get off these anxious stressed trains of thought to arrive at the beautiful quaint village at the next station that we could have enjoyed.

All of these fearful illusions get stored in our subconscious mind, which is actually running the show. Our subconscious minds are the man behind the curtain. However, as soon as we become aware of this man, also known as our ego minds, we are like Dorothy, from the classic 1939 film Wizard of Oz, pulling back the curtain to reveal the seemingly all-powerful flabbergasted Wizard man, attempting to compose himself as he is caught in the façade of pulling the strings of Dorothy's experiences. Like this Wizard, who helps Dorothy realize her *Satnam* or true self, our ego minds can become less invasive and more persuasive to non-fear-based ideologies and uplifting ways of being. Observing our thoughts is a very powerful way of diffusing the power the ego has over our lives and allowing our higher, true selves an opportunity for expression. Yoga is mindfulness. It is letting go and releasing into the moment. Yoga is a practice of expanding who we think we are in order to reveal who we truly are.

"People don't realize that now is all there ever is;
there is no past or future except as memory or anticipation
in your mind."
– *The Power of Now* by Echart Tolle

God grant me the serenity
to accept the things I cannot change;
the courage to change the things I can;
and the wisdom to know the difference. -Alcoholics
Anonymous Prayer

The body also has its own memory contained in each organ and muscle, sometimes called muscle memory. By practicing and breathing into the poses, we create space for the body to heal and to release old habits and emotions that no longer serve our well-being.

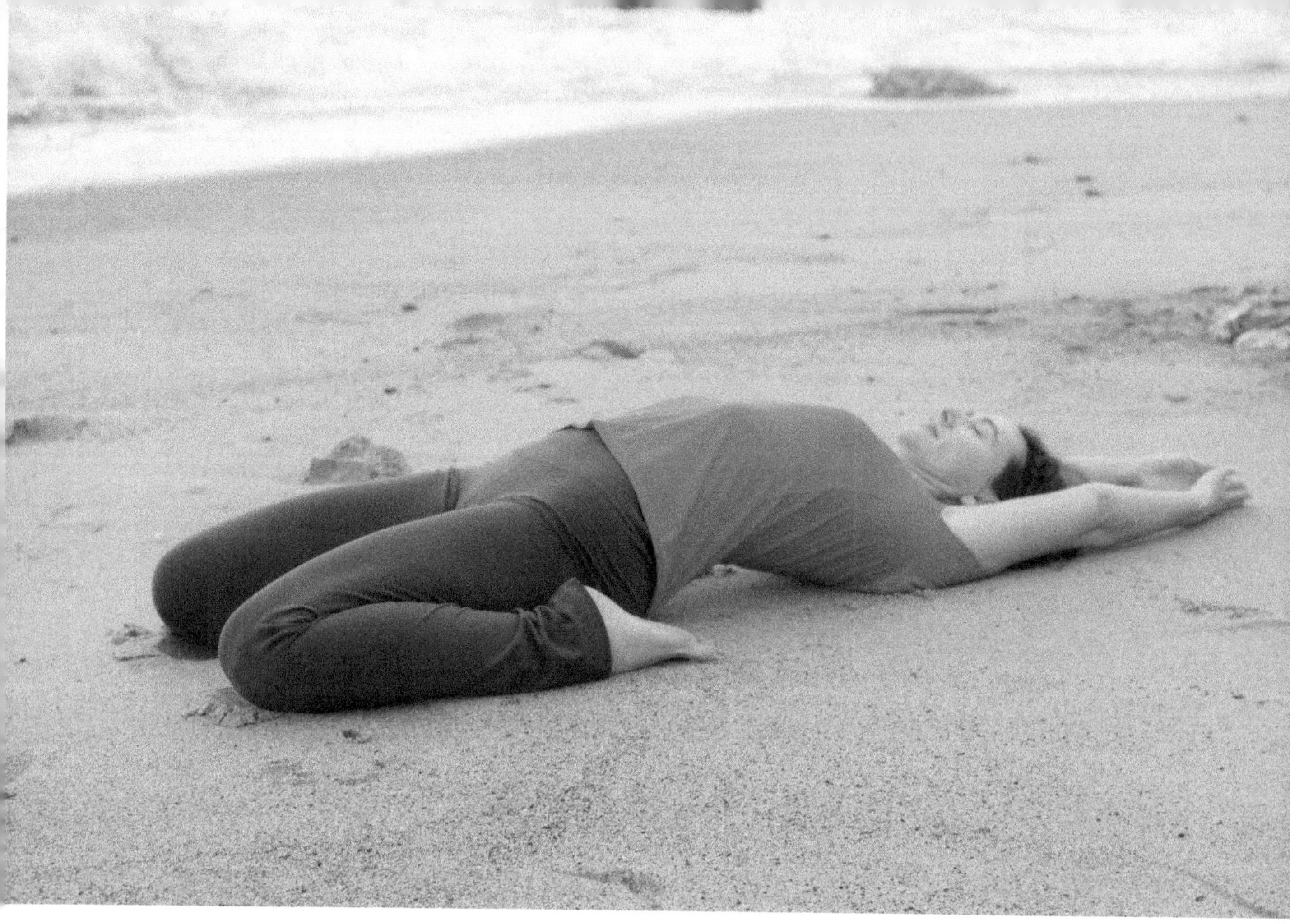

Relaxing in Reclining Warrior Pose, *Supta Virasana*

Releasing all judgement and fear, and breathing into the warrior, gently whispering to relax into the earth, is a way to instantly bring about calm strength that is our true identity.

Benefits

I have created this series, not only, for those who are just beginning or simply want some easy yoga poses to do throughout their day, but also for the more advanced but busy practitioners who require challenges yet efficiency in their practice. Some of these poses may seem overly simple, but if you practice them, they will have tremendous benefits. Yogi Bajan says that we are as young as our spines are flexible. Each of these poses is designed to wake up the Kundalini, a wellspring of potential energy that lies dormant at the base of our spines.

Through the practice of yoga, a practitioner also benefits not only the health of the spine, which is connected to the entire body, but also the joints, nerves, organs, and muscles that are intertwined. Some poses benefit the liver, while others focus on the pituitary gland. All forms of physical exercise have other benefits to the body; for instance, walking stimulates the lymph system. Yoga is not only physical exercise; it is a scientific form of moving the body to benefit the physical, mental and spiritual well-being of humans. Whether you believe in spirituality or not, makes no difference; you can still have a healthy back, body, and mind which can lead ultimately to a more joyful life.

The benefits to specific poses will be listed in the following chapters or weeks as this book is organized. The general benefits of, for example, twists are not only to move the joints of the spine and stretch the muscles but also to massage digestive organs as you breathe deeply into the poses. Balancing poses create a more focused mind, but they can also help to keep you more centered and less likely to fall as you age. They are also challenging, as they require a clear mind to maintain. In addition, balancing poses build confidence and trust in your amazing body and life.

Even though this practice is non-denominational, if this is your desire, you may find the spiritual, either a deepening of your personal spiritual practice or a discovery of one that works for you. I am certain that by honoring myself and through this practice of raising my vibrational energy, I have been led to my own personal spiritual practice. As I grew from a child who said prayers at night into one who questioned the violence and antics of the known world religions, I lost hope that a daily practice would be revealed to me. My only hope, I believed, was to live in a monastery away from the world of violence and temptation. Yoga, like my Buddhist practice, has taught me to be present with the chaos and the order of the world without judgment. This was a big step in finding the spirit of my true self.

How to Use this Book

Each week's lesson comes with an introduction, which explains why I chose that sequence and the benefits of those poses. To experience more amazing benefits of this six week and ultimately lifetime of yoga, also practice the suggestions for "upon waking" and "before bed." I encourage you to practice these rituals and continue even after you have completed the six weeks of yoga routines in this book. If you already have a successful ritual, please continue, or incorporate a little of both. Life is an experience and an experiment.

This six-week program is designed for you to do the routines for a full week at a time. On days when you have a yoga class to attend, you may want to skip that day. Otherwise, to experience the benefits of this simple ten-minute a day practice, I recommend practicing every day.

A great benefit about ten-minutes a day is that even serious athletes, who run every day or swim daily, can add these simple routines into their busy schedules. These ten minutes might just benefit everything else you do in your day, including preparing for that marathon.

Even your work can be enhanced by a yoga practice. If you manage a company, work as a waitress, sit at desk all day writing books, or sing in a rock and roll band, you can benefit from a more flexible, stronger body and the clarity of mind that comes with focusing on the poses and the breath.

Finally, be kind to yourself; do what you can do. The lessons become increasingly more challenging over time. If any pose or modification is too difficult, or if you have knee or joint problems, skip that pose and move on. I will list some modifications for people with specific injuries. But if something feels wrong, and you know it, don't continue that pose. For instance, if you have had a knee surgery, be especially careful with bent knee poses. Also, all practitioners should vigilantly follow the instructions for proper alignment.

However, if, for instance, your hamstrings are tight and Janu Sirsasana, bent knee forward bend, is difficult, if you keep your back straight, you should continue to breathe into this pose. Tight muscles will release with the breath, and weak muscles will become stronger with effort. The key is finding balance and being centered in your practice, not in the antithesis of yoga, overdoing and causing stress because you are unable to fully realize a posture. Being in the moment and breathing into where you are at this precious time is more important.

When you have finished the six weeks, congratulate yourself, and start the program over. You can also skip around to your favorite weeks once you've finished. In the last section, I include suggestions for creating your own ten-minute program and a section of some of my favorite recipes for healthy living. For those who desire more yoga knowledge, enhancing their Bakti Yoga practice, I have included a detailed bibliography and suggested reading section and a more comprehensive list of possible morning and evening affirmations.

For a deeper challenge, I have included a 1.5-hour lesson based on all the postures you've learned over the last six weeks. When you finish the first six weeks, I recommend that you incorporate this session into your schedule to do at least once a week. You can incorporate more of these precious ten-minute sessions into your day, morning, midday, and evening, for instance.

At some point in your practice, if you are lagging in motivation, remember that yoga is a process. There is no end-result. It's a joyous, invigorating, healthy, beautiful, spiritual daily practice that can transform, not only your life, but the lives of all practitioners, and ultimately the world. It is a non-violent way to create more peace, not only in our own lives, but by being living examples for others, we are transforming the world with every breath we take, with every kind word we say, with every wise decision we make for the betterment of ourselves, our families, our communities, and, ultimately, all of humanity and all living beings on this precious, beautiful planet.

Change of any kind comes about by the little things we do every day. That is how we make a big splash or impact in the world. By dipping into the world of peace for ourselves every day, we can create more peace for everyone.

Eat healthy, move freely, breathe deeply, live passionately. Use these ten minutes a day to cleanse the mind of negativity and take a giant step towards your true, amazing selves. Smile just because. Listen with love and express kindness, not only to others, but also to yourself. Feel with all your heart as you open the chest in Cobra Pose. Relax into Savasana as you relax into your beautiful life.

Daily Ritual

UPON WAKING

❈ Practice some or all of these suggestions.

❈ Write in a daily gratitude journal or list silently to yourself five things you are grateful for. Give thanks.

❈ Look in the mirror into your eyes and say, "I am powerful. I am beautiful. I deserve infinite love and abundance. I am healthy." These are only suggestions; you can use your favorite affirmations instead. If this seems a bit silly, remember that being silly is okay. My father used to look in the mirror as he was combing his hair and say, "Handsome devil aren't you." He'd smile, and I could see his confidence building. But as a child I'd laugh and say, "Oh Dad." For some people affirmations or even thinking positively can be as challenging as physical exercise. For this reason, it is beneficial to do this exercise to see what you experience in the process. Also, because many people are also daily bombarded with bad news via magazines in the checkout lines and news reports on the television, radio, and Internet, taking a few moments to counter the negative can yield previously unimaginable positive results. I'm not advocating ignoring the world completely, but rather, finding balance in an imperfect but amazing world by exploring new experiences and possibilities.

❈ Sit for a minute or two and listen to your breath. Listen to your thoughts and say to yourself, "Thinking thoughts. Thank you, ego, for sharing." When you finish, say a personal prayer for how you would like your day to unfold. Trust, have faith and smile and imagine it is done.

❈ Take moments throughout your day to listen to your breath and be present.

Breathing Exercise (Pranayama)

Take a few moments before you begin your yoga practice to connect to your body and mind through the breath. Begin your practice by rolling out a yoga mat or blanket. You might also want to light a candle. As with an actor finding his character, setting the stage with props and wearing a costume, in this case comfortable clothing, help you to savor these precious moments. After setting the stage for your practice, sit comfortably, taking 10 deep breaths, expanding the lower belly first then the middle belly then the upper chest and releasing the lower belly first by gently squeezing the air out by tucking the lower belly in and up towards the rib cage. Think of how we squeeze a tube of toothpaste. If you prefer to exhale opposite of how you inhaled, chest, middle, and then lower belly, if you squeeze as much air out and inhale as much air in, you are practicing Complete Yogic Breath or three-part breathing. If you think of the breath as a flow and not an effort, this exercise will become more natural.

Finding a safe, quiet place to practice sitting meditation, a place where you will not be disturbed, is best. However, you can practice meditation almost anywhere. Because of the current popularity of yoga, I sometimes see practitioners in the park with their eyes closed, looking completely relaxed while sitting on benches or on blankets under the canopy of trees.

By performing Complete Yogic Breath, breathing deeply with intention, you are supplying your body and brain with even more oxygen. As a result, you are also relieving stress by infusing the body with more precious oxygen than the typical shallow breathing often associated with our fast-paced modern society. Shallow or military style breathing is also the "fight or flight" stress creating breath. As stress is one of the main causes of all illnesses, breathing exercises should be part of everyone's preventative care and healing rituals.

Notice how you are breathing throughout your day. When you are experiencing stress, take a moment to focus on the breath, breathing deeply into the lower belly. Count ten healing breaths and see if you do not feel a little lighter and less stressed.

Before Bed

❀ Avoid energizing, or stressful activities. I witnessed the stress that watching negative news or violent programs just before bed many years ago with roommates and with myself. I realized that these activities could cause the very stress that I was working in my yoga and mindfulness practices to alleviate. Resisting the temptation to look at computers and phone screens is also a good idea because, not only the content on them, but the lights on the screens can interfere with our sleep.

❀ Review your day and list five things you are grateful for.

❀ Ask your body, mind, and spirit for a deep restful sleep.

❀ Imagine how you want your day to flow for the next day.

❀ And relax in the awareness that your request has already been granted.

❀ Smile and close your eyes, knowing that tomorrow will be even more vibrant and abundant than today.

GOOD NIGHT... *Namaste.*

"It's not about "having time; it's about making time."

WEEK ONE

INTRO

Congratulate yourself! You bought the book. You've committed to an amazing journey. You are here! Every time we commit to our own growth, we are becoming the change we want to see in the world.

"Your time is limited, so don't waste it living someone else's life." – Steve Jobs

DHARMA

Are you willing to lose yourself to find yourself? There may be no absolutes in the world or magic potions. However, one thing is for certain, the answers and questions that will lead us both as individuals and collectively to our true divine selves lie in the "constellations of our hearts."

There are many questions in life, and science and logic cannot answer them all. However, perhaps the combination of the magic of three, science, logic and love can solve those problems. And what if the body is love incarnate, a mystical living vessel of love?

❀ Science (the body)

❀ Logic (the mind)

❀ Love (the soul)

PHYSICAL EXERCISE – 10 MINUTES OR 108 BREATHS (*VINYASA*)

Move gently between poses. There's no need to rush. Breathe through the nose unless otherwise specified. Savor each pose, making this the longest ten minutes of your life.

TADASANA, MOUNTAIN POSE

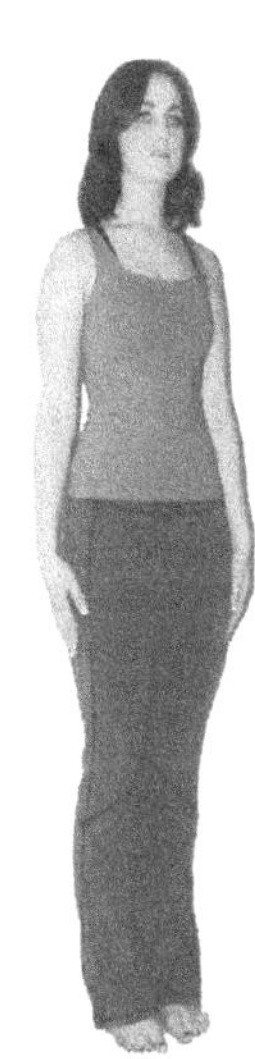

Stand centered with the toes spread evenly, the big toes together, and the heels slightly apart, and lift the arches of the feet. The legs are straight and strong but resist locking the knees. Internally rotate the thighs and tuck the sitting bones under. Relax the shoulders while you lift the chest and imagine a string pulling the crown of your head up as energy flows from the earth through your feet to the crown of your head and out. Stand for a few moments inhaling energy from the earth and the sky and exhaling back to the earth and the sky. You could inhale from the sky and exhale to the earth and then reverse, becoming the conduit between the two. Hold *Tadasana*, as strong as a mountain, for 5-10-breaths.

Benefits

Tadasana strengthens the abdomen, legs, and arches of the feet. It may help relieve sciatica and foot pain associated with sinking arches. You can practice this pose anywhere. Waiting in line at the supermarket is now an opportunity to stretch taller and breathe deeper.

SIDE BENDS

Stand with the feet a little more than hip-width distance apart and inhale center. The arms are comfortably raised, and elbows bent (Position A.)

Remember to stretch the spine long and keep the head neutral. Again, maintain internal rotation of the thighs as in *Tadasana*. Exhale as you bend to the side, using the arm on the opposite side to support the body into bending deeply (Position B.)

Let the head relax and hang. Continue flowing as you breathe, taking deep breaths, inhaling center, and exhaling to the side. Focus on the breath and the movement, stretching the entire length of the body, releasing on each side 10-20-breaths.

Benefits

Side Bends stretch and strengthen the entire side of the body and warm and lubricate the joints of the back, hips, shoulders, and neck. And a bonus is that it is great for love handles.

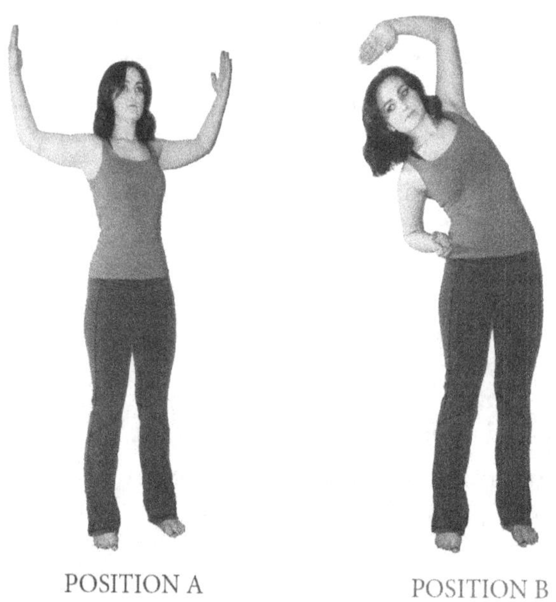

POSITION A   POSITION B

FORWARD BEND FLOW

Stand with the feet hip-width distance apart, the toes slightly pointing in, and lift the arches of the feet. Continue to maintain internal rotation of the thighs. Inhale while circling the arms around the body. As your hands come together in prayer pose above your head, look-up and arch back, (Position A.)

Exhale and fold forward with the strength of the legs, bending the knees as necessary to place the palms on the floor (Position B.)

If you cannot reach the floor comfortably, you may place your palms on blocks (Position C) or a chair.

Continue flowing as you breathe, again focusing on your breath and the movements 10-20-breaths.

Benefits

The first two poses of the Sun Salutation are a great way to practice gentle back bending and re-aligning the spine. This flow relieves tension in the lower back and stretches and strengthens the calf and the hamstring muscles along the back of the legs, which connect to the lower back and help protect the back from injury.

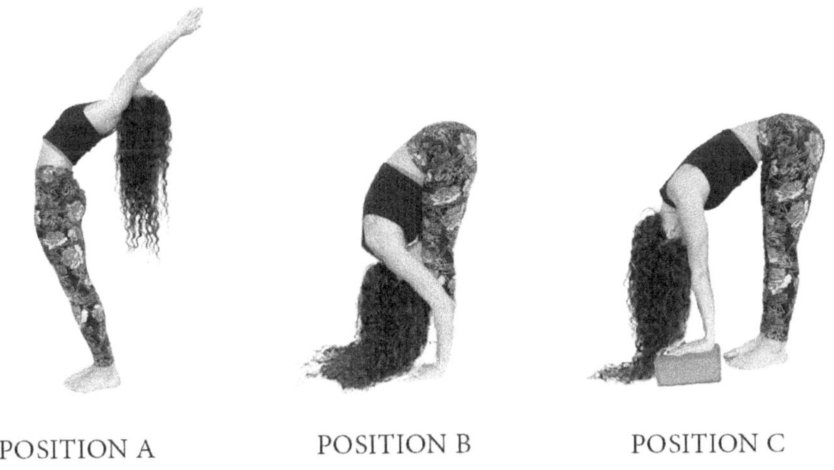

POSITION A   POSITION B   POSITION C

STANDING FORWARD BEND, *PASCHIMOTTANASANA*

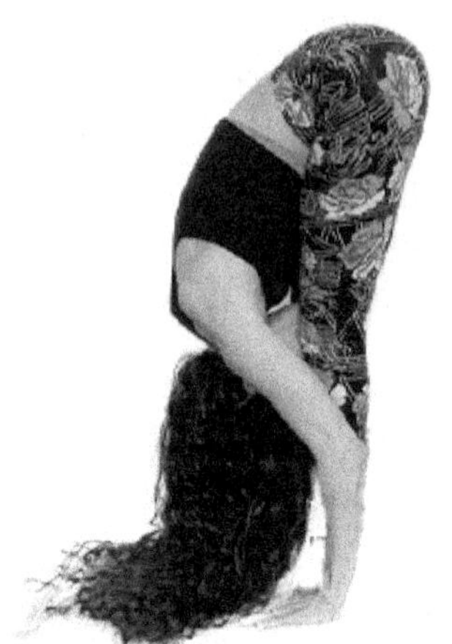

Exhale, performing one more forward bend flow. As you release, if you cannot reach the floor, hold the elbows and hang, lifting the sitting bones while relaxing the back. With each breath imagine releasing a little more. The weight is centered over the feet with the toes slightly pointing inward. Again, maintain internal rotation of the thighs and allow the back to release gently. Let the head, neck, and spine hang like a vine hanging from a branch on a tree. Take 5-10 deep breaths. Then Inhale and gently roll up to standing.

Benefits

Paschimottanasana is a complete stretch from the back of the head to the heels, particularly stretching the hamstrings while releasing tension in the entire spine. This pose also massages the internal digestive organs and has been known to relieve constipation, sciatica and invigorate the nervous system.

"Everything depends on what is in our hearts. If we decide to our-selves that something is impossible, then, consistent with our minds in thinking so, even something that is possible for us will become impossible. On the other hand, if we have the confidence that we can definitely do something, then we are already one step closer to achieving it in reality."
– Daisaku Ikeda

SHOULDER ROLLS

Begin by rolling the shoulders in big circles. Do 5-10, rolling up, back, down and forward (Position A).

Then do the reverse direction, rolling up, forward, down, and back (Position B).

Benefits

Shoulder rolls relieve tension held in shoulders, lubricate joints, and stretch shoulder muscles. By releasing tension in the shoulders, allowing more blood to flow to the neck and head, this pose can also help relieve and alleviate headaches.

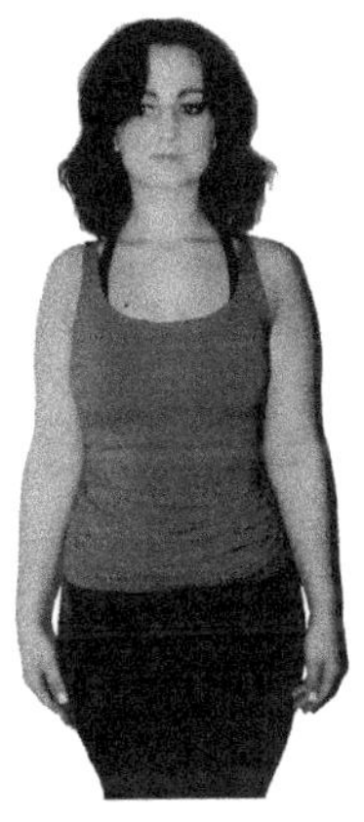

POSITION A

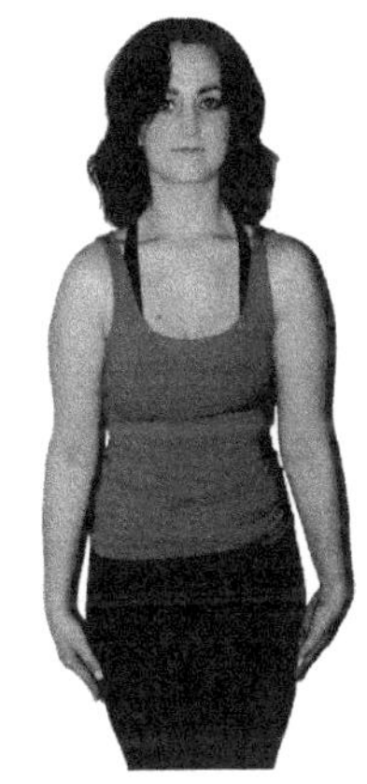

POSITION B

The shoulders are where we keep much of our daily stress. When the trapezius muscles along the back of the shoulders become stressed and tight, they can constrict blood flow to the neck and head causing neck pain and headaches. This is a great exercise to do throughout the day, especially for office workers who tend to pinch their shoulders as they type on computers. See the section on ergonomics for more information on proper posture while sitting at a desk.

GENTLE NECK ROLLS

Inhale the head straight up as if a string is pulling the crown of the head up (Position A).

Exhale, release the chin to the chest. Then Inhale back to center. Exhale, releasing the left ear towards the left shoulder (Position B).

Inhale back to center. Exhale, release the neck gently back (Position C).

Do not allow the neck to flop back or over stretch. Use the neck muscles to control the stretch and resist the temptation to squinch the shoulders up. Instead, gently release the shoulders away from the ears. Inhale back to center. Exhale the right ear to the right shoulder. Continue until you have done at least 3-5 in each position.

Benefits

Neck rolls relieve tension held in the neck muscles, lubricate the vertebrae, stretch the shoulder muscles and so much more.

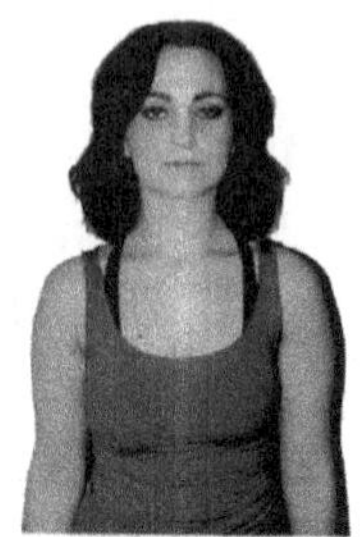

POSITION A

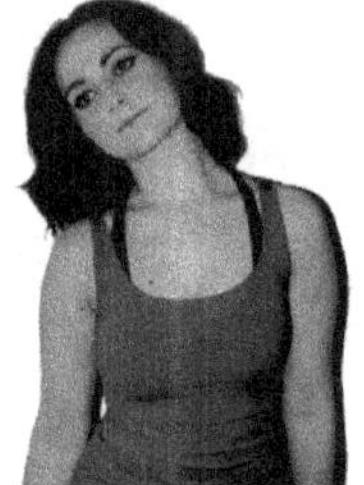

POSITION B

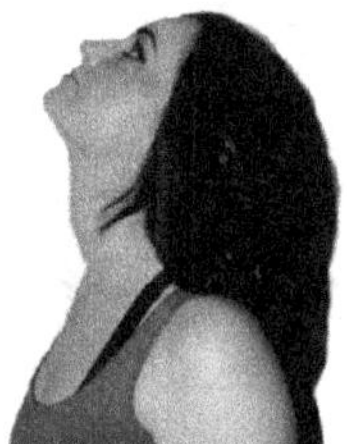

POSITION C

According to the National Institute of Health, "Neck pain is an important personal and societal burden, affecting 30% to 50% of adults in the general population in any given year." Because neck pain is so prevalent and often debilitating, it is essential to do all that we can to heal properly and to maintain health in all parts of our spines, cervical, thoracic, and lumbar equally.

CAT / COW POSE

Exhale onto the hands and knees with the hands under the shoulders, and the knees under the hips. Inhale and lift the head, chest and sitting bones while releasing the middle back to sink down like a cow (Position A).

Exhale and drop the head while tucking the sitting bones under and rounding the back up like a scared cat (Position B).

Stretch and breathe deeply in each pose for 10-20-breaths.

Benefits

Cat / Cow Pose warms the body, stimulates the nervous system, lubricates the joints in the spine, and massages the kidneys. These two poses also strengthen the wrists and arms and are an easy way to safely begin to create healthy flexibility in the spine.

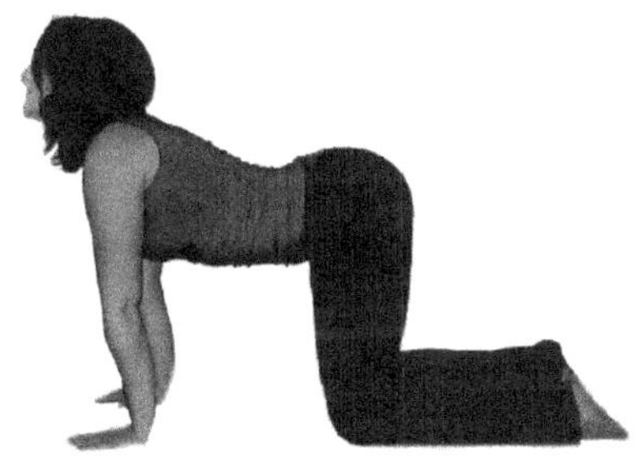

POSITION A

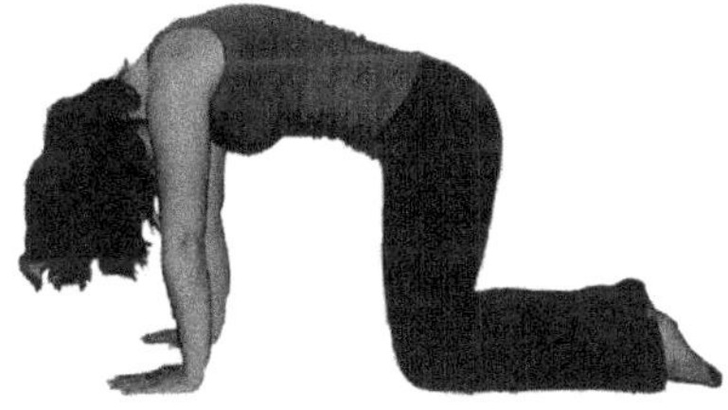

POSITION B

EXTENDED CHILD'S POSE, *GARBHASANA*

Drop the hips to the heels of the feet. Knees are a little more than hip-width distance apart. Drop the chest towards the ground and spread the fingers reaching forward. Relax the forehead to the floor. The arms are extended straight out with relaxed elbows. Do not force. Let the breath release you into the pose gently. Stretch the top of the spine forward while stretching the lower back towards the heels. If you have any discomfort in the knees, sit on a pillow to modify the pose. You may also place a pillow under the chest for support. Relax and breathe into the lower back – 5-10 long breaths.

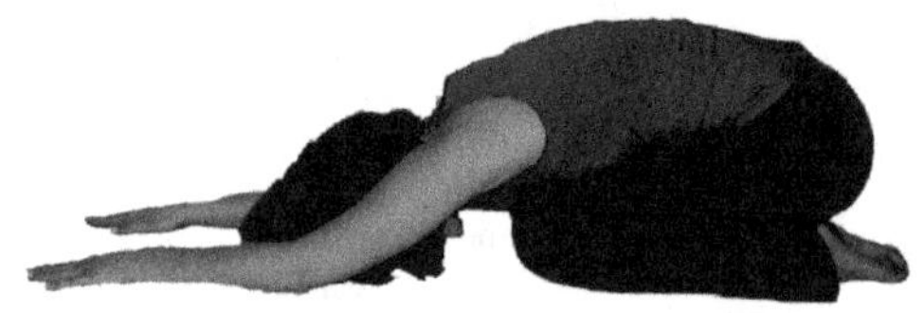

The descriptions and images are guides to help you reach for the appropriate posture. If you cannot reach your head to the floor at this time, simply breathe and relax the hips and joints of the spine and neck, breathing deeply into the lower back.

Benefits

Garbhasana relieves pressure in the spine, strengthens and stretches the quadriceps, the abductor muscles, the hips, and lower back, and stretches from the fingertips to the sitting bones. This pose can also help relieve tension in the shoulders.

STAFF POSE, *DANDASANA*

Transition from Child's Pose by sliding the legs from under you and place them straight in front, making a 90-degree angle with the body and legs. This pose looks deceivingly easy. Performed properly, it is a very challenging pose. Sit on a pillow if your back is rounded. Stretch the back tall and straight using the abdominal and back muscles. Lift the chest. Ground the legs into the earth and stretch from the heels outward. Slightly tuck your chin and place the palms on the ground near your hips. Breathe deeply for 5-breaths.

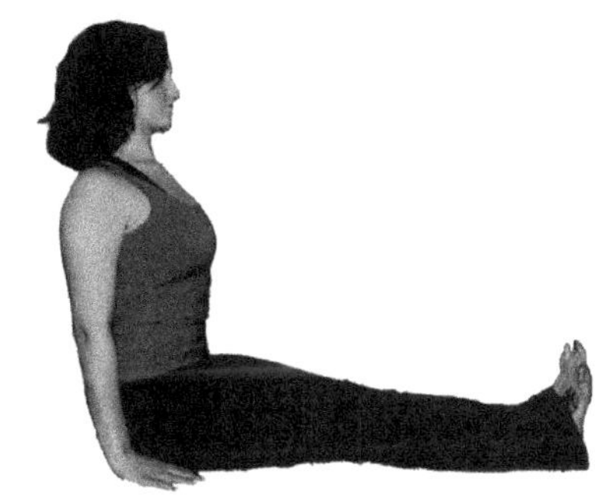

Benefits

Dandasana reduces fat around the waistline, tones the kidneys and stretches and strengthens the entire back of the body.

BENT KNEE, MODIFIED *ARDHA NAVASANA*

Bend the knees, place the soles of feet on the floor, and straighten the arms. Lean back in a gentle 45-degree angle, engage the abdominal muscles, and gaze forward. The palms should hover a few inches away from the outside of the knees. Hug the knees and relax for a breath in between repetitions. Hold each posture for 5 long breaths. Repeat 3-5 times. Return to Dandasana.

Benefits

Ardha Navanansana strengthens the abdominal and lower back muscles and tones the liver, gall bladder and spleen. This modified pose also prepares the body for the full pose and other more advanced postures.

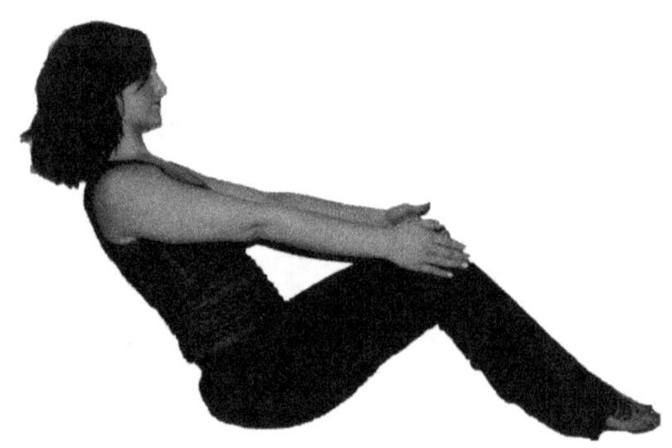

"The importance of having a healthy lower back can be realized if we watch old people when they sit down, get up and walk. Consciously or unconsciously, they support their backs with their hands. This indicates that the back is weak and cannot withstand the strain. As long as the back is strong and needs no support, one feels young though advanced in age. This asana brings life and vigor to the back and enables us to grow old gracefully and comfortably." – Light On Yoga by B.K.S. Iyengar.

Sit and straighten the right leg and place the left foot on the right side of the right knee. Center your left hand, facing back, about a foot behind you, wrap your right arm around your left knee and begin to twist the lower, middle, then upper back to the left as you turn the head to gaze behind you. Twist a little more with each exhale. Take 5-breaths and repeat on the other side. Return to Dandasana between poses.

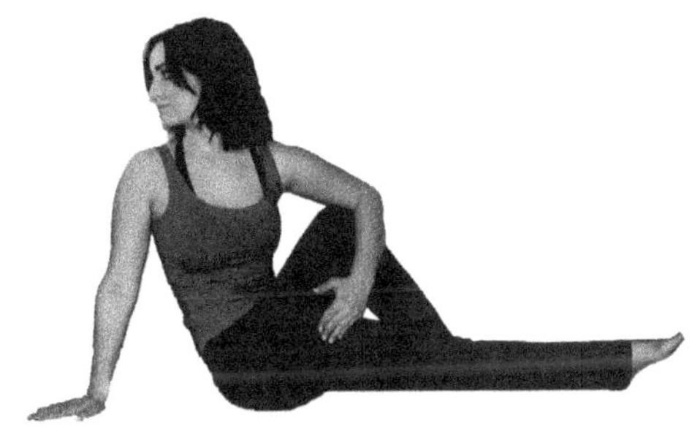

Benefits

Twist along with back bends are the best poses for invigorating and maintaining the flexibility of the spine. While you breathe deeply, this pose also massages internal organs.

RELAXATION POSE, *SAVASANA*

Lie back, extending the legs straight, letting the feet hang open. Place your arms a comfortable distance from your sides with the palms facing up. Close the eyes and relax. Focus on the breath and inhale into any tension you still feel in the body. Then release this tension as you exhale. Imagine filling your body completely, down to your fingertips and toes, as if the body were a balloon. Then release into the earth as you exhale, completely relaxing, knowing you are supported in all your endeavors. Watch any thoughts that come into the mind and release them without judgment, letting these thoughts float away on a cloud. Relax for at least 10 - 30 long deep breaths, 5 - 10 minutes is best if you have time.

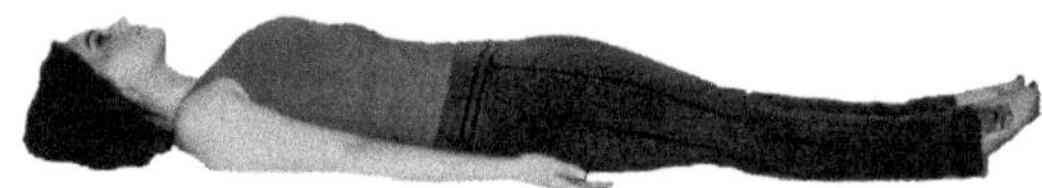

Come out of *Savasana* gently. Open the eyes with a soft gaze, turning the head as you exhale to the right side, inhale center, and then exhale to the left. Take another long breath and roll onto your side in a fetal position and inhale up to sitting when you are ready.

You may want to skip this part of the exercise, *Savasana*, but it is the icing on the cake for your practice. In this divine stillness the body can incorporate the benefits of the postures you have just performed.

Benefits

Savasana is perhaps the most important pose in yoga. These moments of stillness and complete relaxation allow the body to incorporate the benefits of all the other postures of yoga. It also creates a calmness of the mind and prepares the body for meditation and the realization of the oneness of creation.

Sit comfortably for a moment then bow to your higher self, your true self, the universe, and or God, whatever you choose that brought you to this wonderful day and say "Namaste," which means, "The god in me honors the god in you."

HAVE A BLESSED DAY, NAMASTE

Releasing our recorded limitations that plague our minds
with past and future fears, creating resentment, worry,
and unhealthy stress, involves, first, viewing our thoughts
as an outside non-judgmental observer, then allowing
these thoughts to float away peacefully so that we may
return through the awareness of our breath to the present
moment. Reciting a mantra or simply sitting and focusing
on the breath for a few moments leaves our minds clean
and fresh for our day.

I think of my meditation and chanting practices as brushing and flossing my teeth. If we want to keep our teeth, we take care of them and keep them clean of old consumptions. In the case of our teeth, these are the foods and drinks we previously ingested. In the same way, we can keep our minds clean of old consumptions, the ideas, events, fears, desires etc. that we have previously consumed. This way we are cleaning our minds of clutter, so that we may embody the clarity to create a brighter future for ourselves, those we love, and ultimately all of humanity.

Week One Summary of Poses

TADASANA OR MOUNTAIN –
5 Breaths
SIDE BENDS - 10 Breaths

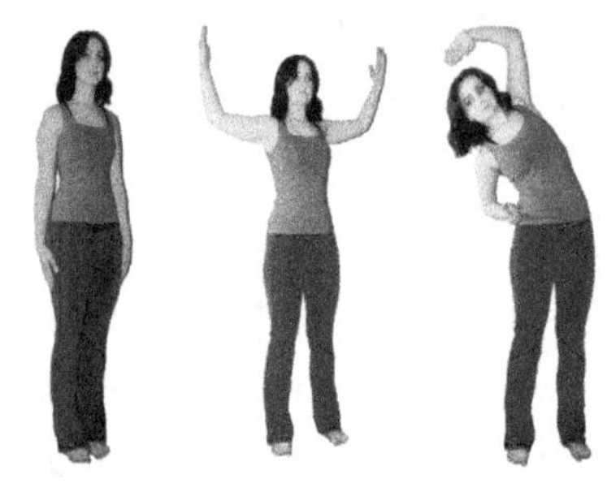

FORWARD BEND FLOW –
10 Breaths
STANDING FORWARD BEND –
5 Breaths

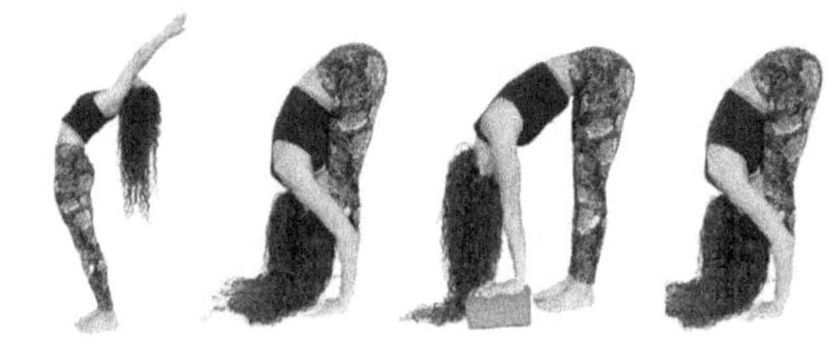

SHOULDER ROLLS –
5 Breaths forward and 5 Breaths
back
NECK ROLLS – 3 Breaths roll right
and 3 Breaths roll left

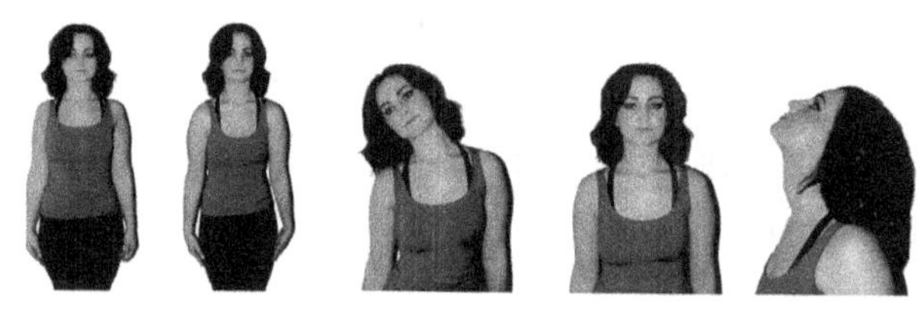

CAT / COW POSES – 10 Breaths
EXTENDED CHILD'S POSE –
5 Breaths

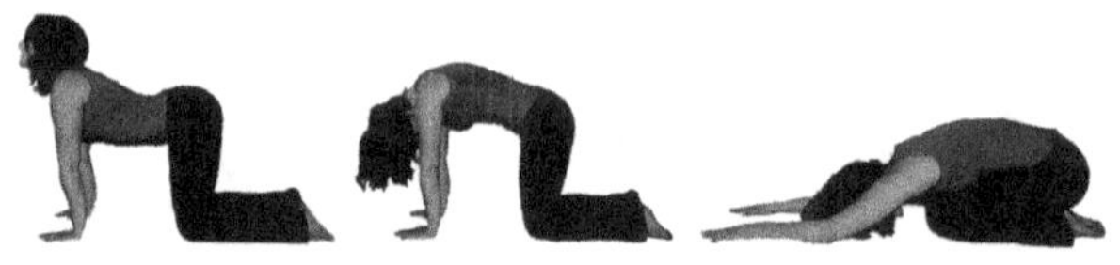

DANDANSA OR STAFF POSE –
5 Breaths
MODIFIED BOAT POSE –
5 Breaths X 3

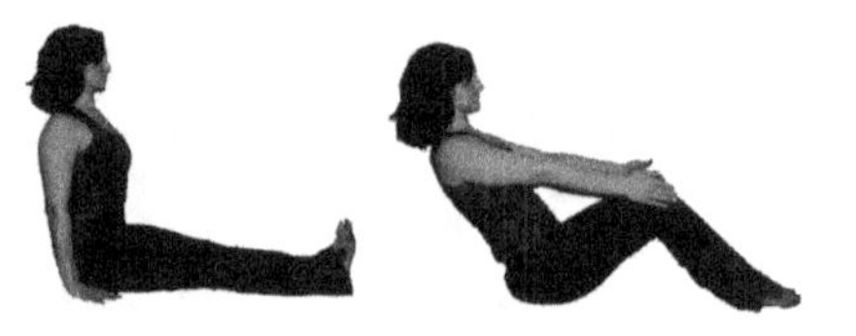

SEATED TWIST – 10 Breaths
SAVASANA OR RELAXATION POSE
– 10 TO 20 Breaths

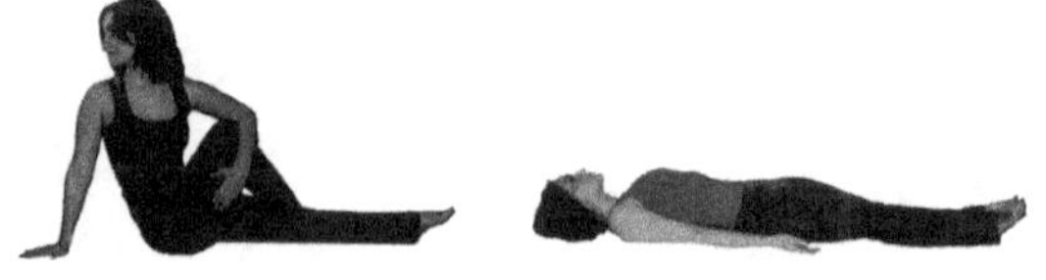

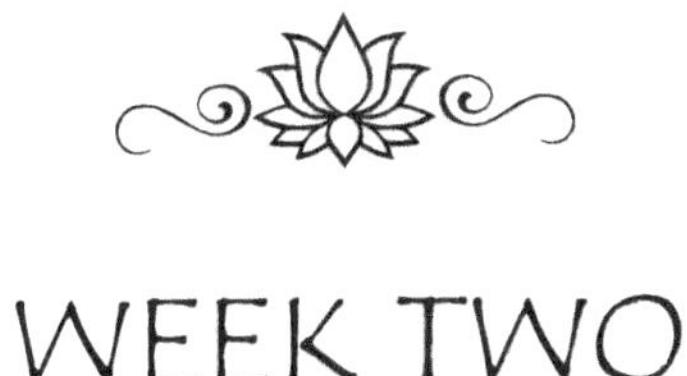

WEEK TWO

INTRO

This week's lesson is designed to invigorate the spine, warm and detoxify the body, and continue the process of exploring the possibilities of breath and movement that are yoga. And through this union of body, breath, and soul, may you embark on the greatest journey of all, continuing to explore the possibilities of self-discovery.

DHARMA

Love of oneself can be the greatest love of all; it is from this place that all love must emerge. Without it, there is nothing to give. Nurturing our own growth is not a selfish act, but rather a selfless act. When we are full of energy and grace, we can impart that which we have been given and nurtured unto the world. Who could deny that the world needs all of us to be functioning at our best?

Asana practice could be regarded as a form of
asceticism, a way of transcending the body. Or the
practice could be viewed as a way of daily rejoicing in
what is - strong, flexible, supple, and amazing.

BREATHING EXERCISES (PRANAYAMA)

BREATH OF FIRE, *AGNI-PRASANA*

Sit comfortably, inhale deeply, then powerfully release the breath by squeezing the lower belly in and up and exhaling through the mouth making a sound "Ha" as in doing a karate chop. Repeat this several times. Now breathe only through the nose, focusing on exhaling, squeezing the lower belling in and up. Expand the belly as you inhale, letting the lungs fill from this vacuum effect naturally. Breathe in short energetic bursts, pumping the lower belly faster and faster until you create a rhythm that seems never ending. There should be a sound as you exhale powerfully through the nose, 10-20-breaths. Pause then take a deep inhale and exhale. Repeat 2 more times.

Benefits

Breath of Fire is a cleansing, detoxifying breath that creates heat in the body. This breath has many more benefits that you can read about in *Light on Pranayama* by B.K.S. Iyengar.

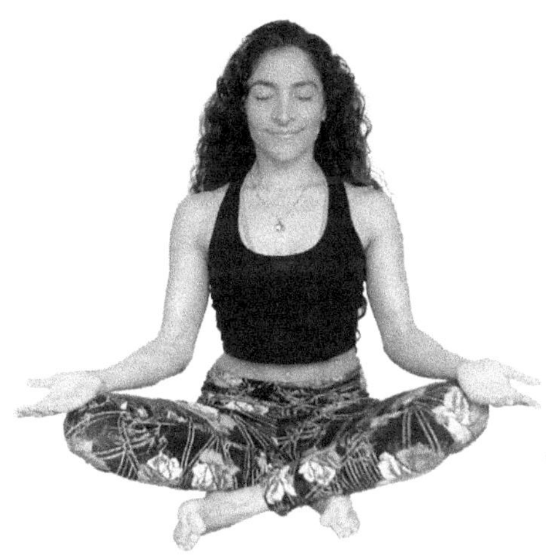

NEW POSES (VINYASA)

Move gently between poses. There's no need to rush. Breathe through the nose unless otherwise specified. You may want to add a blanket under your mat this week for extra padding.

Roll out your mat and sit cross-legged. You may place a pillow under your sitting bones if this is difficult for the knees. Sit with the hands on the knees with palms facing up. Stretch the spine tall, tuck the chin slightly, and imagine a line of energy pulling from the sitting bones up to the crown of the head. Relax the shoulders down and expand the lower belly as you breathe deeply – three-part yogic breath for 5-10-breaths.

Many events happen in life. There are joyous days and times of suffering. Sometimes unpleasant circomstances occur. But that's what makes life so interesting. The dramas we encounter are part and parcel of being human. If we experienced no change or drama in our lives, if nothing unexpected ever happened, we would merely be like automatons, our lives unbearably monotonous and dull. Therefore, please develop a strong self so that you can enact the drama of your life with confidence and poise in the face of whatever vicissitudes you may encounter.

Place the hands on the shins or the knees and hold firmly. Relax the shoulders, inhale and lift the chest and belly, arching the lower and upper back into a C-like position. (Position A). Exhale and release, rounding the spine back (Position B).

Remember this is still an active stretch, so rather than relax as your round the back, focus on stretching as you exhale. Try to keep the head in a neutral position, which will protect the neck from overextending.

Breathe powerfully, focusing your awareness more on the exhale. Move quickly – 10-20-breaths (Breath of Fire optional).

You can do this exercise twice moving the hands from the shins, flexing the lower back, to the knees to flex the middle back.

Benefits

Spine flexes warm the body, gently move the spine, and combined with the breath, are detoxifying for the body. This series also invigorates the nervous system.

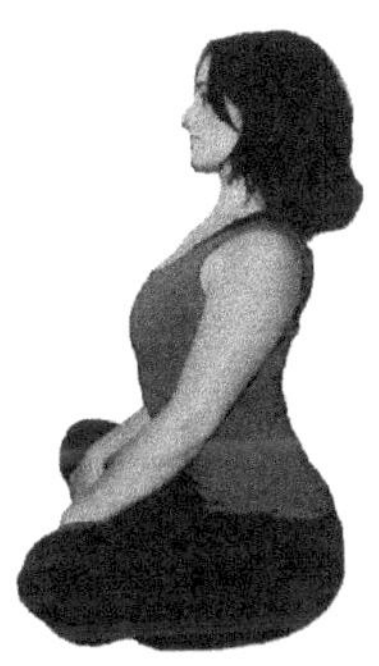

POSITION A

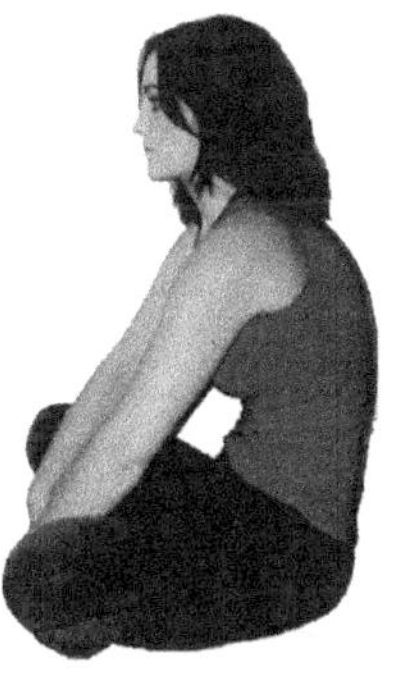

POSITION B

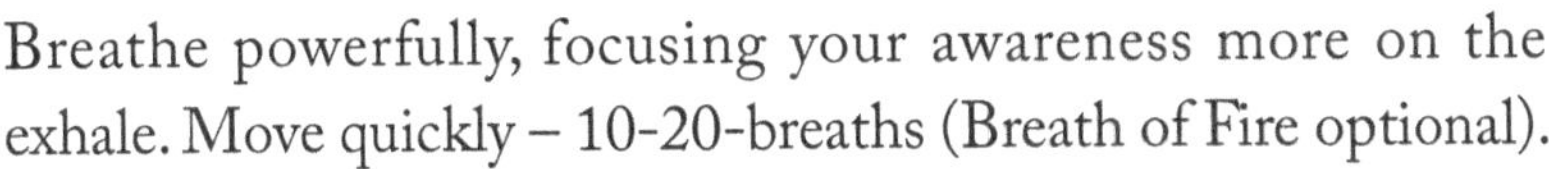

Health is not simply the absence of illness. Real health is the will to overcome every form of adversity and use even the worst of circumstances as a springboard for new growth and development. Simply put, the essence of health is the constant renewal and rejuvenation of life.

WASHING MACHINE

Place the hands on the shoulders with the fingers
facing forward and the thumbs back. Breathe powerfully again focusing on the exhale. Inhale twist to
the left and look behind you, exhale and look right.
Move quickly pumping the lower belly as you breathe
10-20-breaths (Breath of Fire is optional).

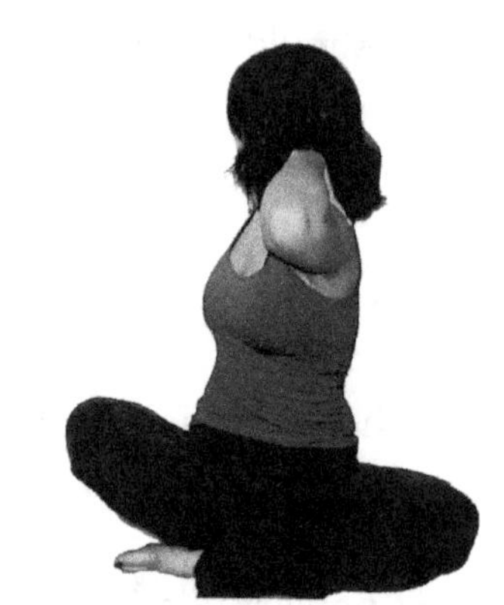

Benefits

Washing Machine lubricates the joints of the spine,
warms the body, helps release tension in the neck, also
detoxifies the body via the breath, and massages internal organs.

SHOULDER DROPS

Inhale lift the shoulders towards the ears. While exhaling let the shoulders drop. The
arms hang loosely by the side. Sitting tall, focusing on exhaling, breathe powerfully for
5-10-breaths.

Benefits

Relieves tension and stress held in the shoulders,
which can help alleviate headaches and free the
shoulders and neck for even more valuable creativity.

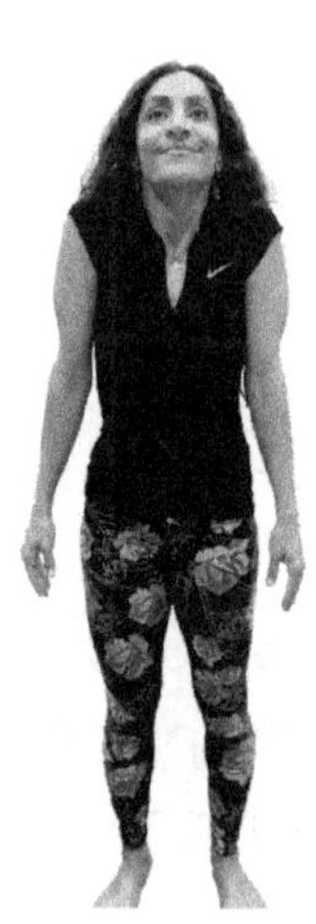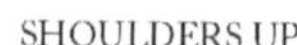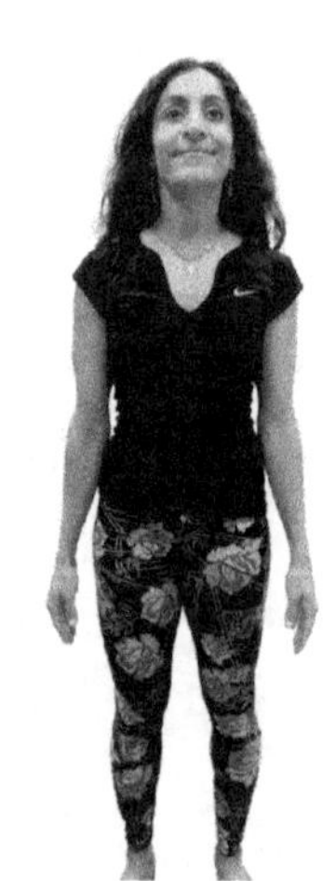

SHOULDERS UP   SHOULDERS DOWN

CROSS-LEGGED FORWARD BEND

While sitting cross-legged, drop the head and reach the arms in front of you. If you cannot place the head on the floor, use a pillow or releaase as far as you can without straining the lower back. Breathe into the lower back and the hips – 5-breaths. Swap the legs and repeat for 5-breaths, breathing into the opposite hip. If this pose is too challenging, you may use a pillow under the sitting bones.

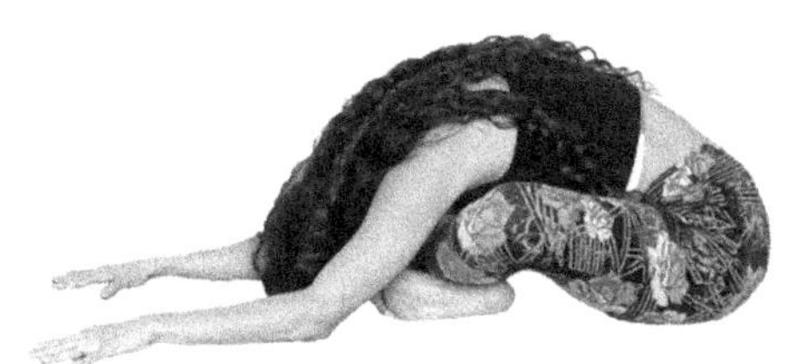

Benefits

Cross-Legged Forward Bend gently stretches the lower back, hips, groin muscles, and the upper back, relieving tension and stress as we breath deeply.

CAT / COW POSE – 10-20 BREATHS *(WEEK ONE)*

"Seeds of past karma cannot germinate if they are roasted in the fires of divine wisdom." "Since you alone are responsible for your thoughts, only you can change them." "Retire to the center of your being, which is calmness." "The wave is the same as the ocean, though it is not the whole ocean."
– Paramahansa Yogananda

BENT KNEE DOWN DOG

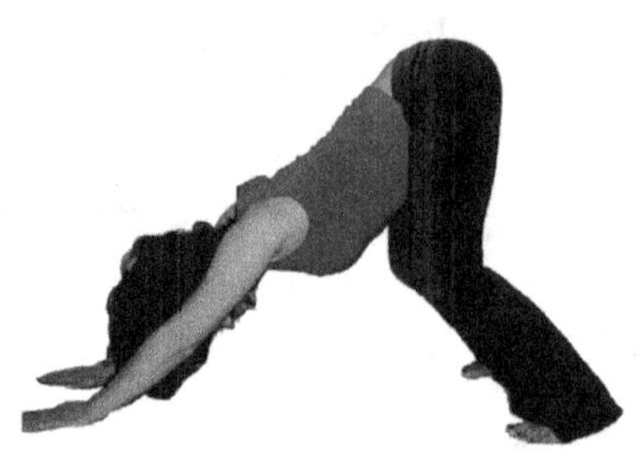

On your last exhale, inhale into cow one more time, exhale, place the feet at the side edges of the mat, bend the knees, and stretch the back. Push the sitting bones back while pressing the floor away with your hands. Keep the knees bent to stretch the spine as much as possible. Relax the neck and drop the head. Gaze between the feet at the floor. While tilting the sitting bones up, imagine a string pulling your chest to the floor for 5-breaths.

Benefits

Bent Knee Down Dog stretches and strengthens the arms, and gently stretches the entire back of the legs to the heels including the hamstring and Achilles tendon. This pose also calms the brain and helps relieve mild depression and stretches and strengthens the shoulders.

EXTENDED CHILD'S POSE – 5-10 LONG BREATHS *(WEEK ONE)*

DANDASANA OR STAFF POSE BREATHE DEEPLY FOR 5-10 BREATHS *(WEEK ONE)*

"Change only happens in the present moment. The past is already done. The future is just energy and intention."
– Kino MacGregor.

BOAT / FORWARD BEND FLOW

From Dandasana, inhale as you engage the abdominal muscles to lean back about 45 degrees and stretch the arms straight out parallel with the shoulders and the ground (Position A).

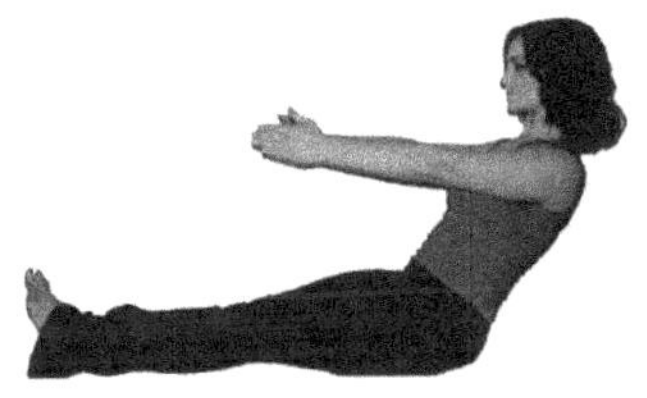

POSITION A

As you exhale, reach the arms forward towards the feet as if holding a ball between your hands (Position B).

Hinge at the hips, keeping the back straight in its natural posture, not rounded. Lift the chest, breathing deeply 10-20-breaths.

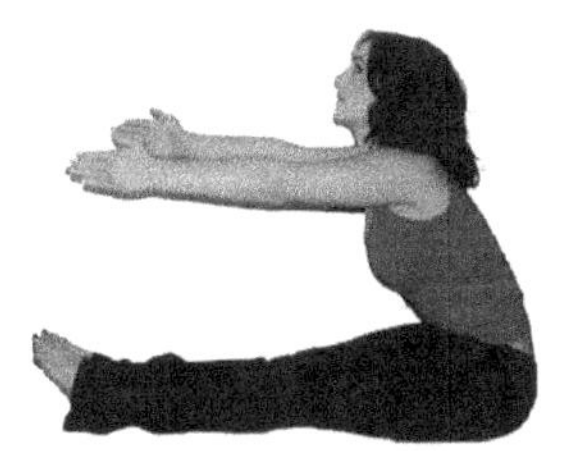

POSITION B

Benefits

This flow strengthens the abdominal area, which helps to protect the back, stretches the hamstring, and invigorates the entire nervous system that runs along the back of the legs. This flow also prepares the body for more advanced postures like forward bends and full Boat Pose, Paripurna Navasana.

"Keep moving forward, even one or two steps, in your own way. Those who live out their lives to the fullest, unperturbed by the noisy clamor around them, are the true winners."
– Daisaku Ikeda

BRIDGE POSE, *SETU BANDHA SARVANGASANA*

Bend the knees, roll the back down to the mat, and place
the feet hip-width distance apart just below the sitting
bones. Relax the arms by your side, inhale and begin to
lift the hips, belly and chest. The shoulders, head and
neck remain on the floor. Stretch more into the pose as if
a string were pulling the middle belly and heart up to the
ceiling. Now if you can, clasp the hands under your back
and push the arms into the mat while lifting the belly
and chest higher. Resist the urge to separate the knees;
keep the legs parallel, 5-10 long deep breaths.

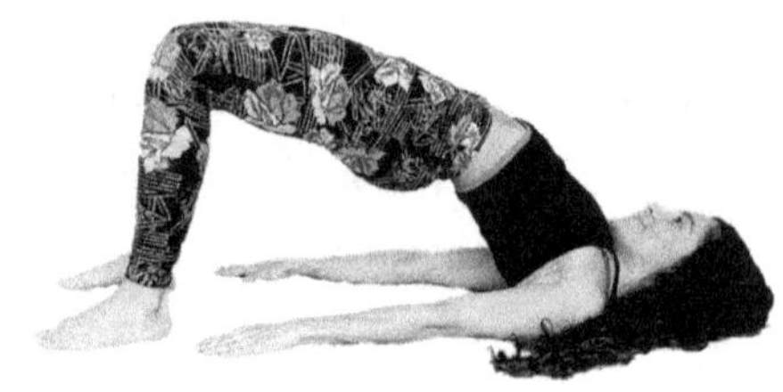

POSITION A

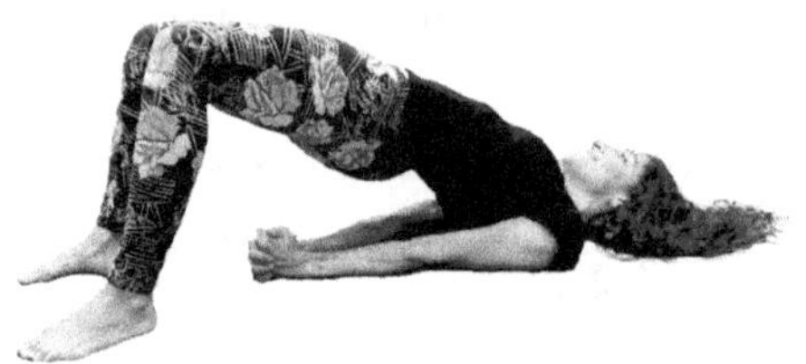

POSITION B

Benefits

Easy Bridge Pose stretches the front of the body, opens the chest, relieves lower back pain
caused by compression, and gently bends and expands the vertebrae of the back creating
space for healing. It also strengthens the quadriceps muscles and the knees. In addition, this
pose is a gentle inversion, good for detoxifying the lungs and draining lymph nodes and
calming the brain of anxiety.

While you stretch in bridge pose, you might imagine that
you are letting go of something you have been holding
onto so that you can cross over to the other side. You are
not only crossing over a bridge, but you are the bridge at
the same time. You are this strong structure spanning two
different sides of an issue or two different ways of living or
two different ways of being. As you cross over to live as
your higher self, you are the bridge that also inspires others
and helps others to discover their own true selves.

SAVASANA

Lie flat with the legs straight and feet a little more than hip-width distance apart. Place your arms a comfortable distance by your side with the palms facing up. Close your eyes and relax. Focus on your breath, inhaling into any tension you still feel in the body while releasing deeper into the pose on each exhale.

Imagine your breath is like an ocean tide. As you inhale, the ocean rises on the shore of your body into the fingertips and toes. As you exhale, the breath slowly returns to the infinite ocean of all that is. Observe any thoughts that come into the mind and release them without judgment, letting them float away. Breathe at least 10-30 long deep breaths, 5-10 minutes is best

This is one of my favorite meditations during Savasana. Connecting to the infinite is an amazing experience, not only for releasing tension and stress that may still mar our minds and bodies, but also for creating more peace in the world by first finding it within.

Follow with a few moments of sitting on a pillow comfortably, breathing deeply. Bow with the hands in prayer saying Namaste, Meaning, "The god in me honors the god in you." You can imagine telling your body this.

HAVE A BLESSED DAY, NAMASTE.

Week Two Summary of Poses

CROSS LEGGED SITTING –
5 Breaths
SPINE FLEXES - 10 Breaths

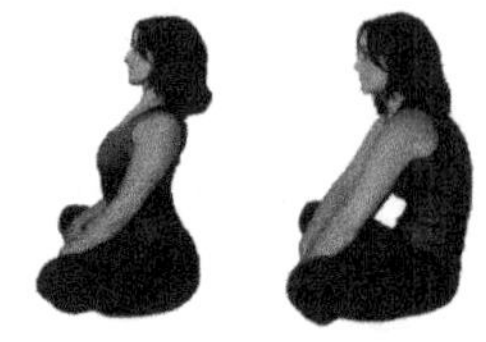

WASHING MACHINE –
10 Breaths
SHOULDER DROPS – 5 Breaths

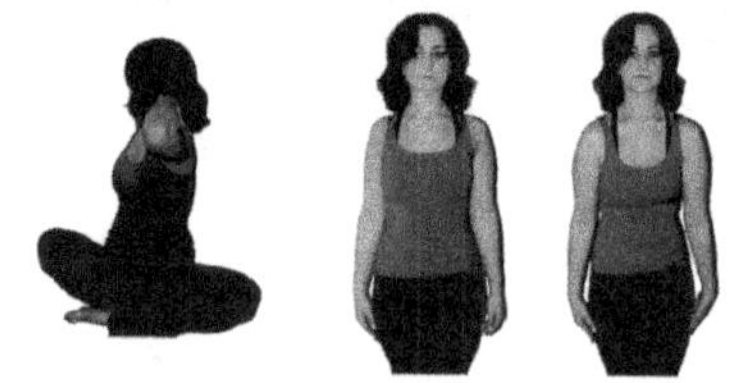

CROSS LEGGED FORWARD BEND –
5 Breaths right leg and 5 Breaths left
CAT / COW POSES – 10 Breaths

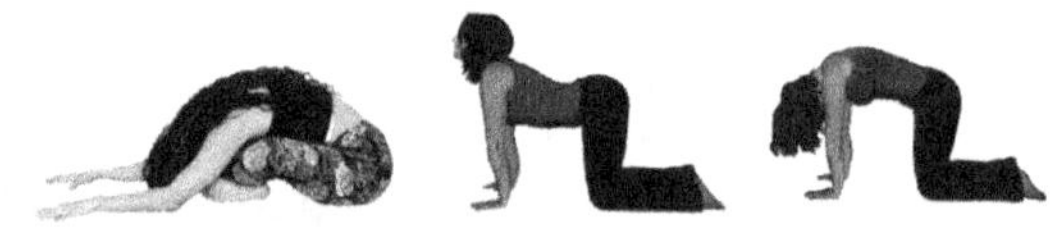

BENT KNEE DOWN DOG –
5 Breaths
EXTENDED CHILD'S POSE –
5 Breaths

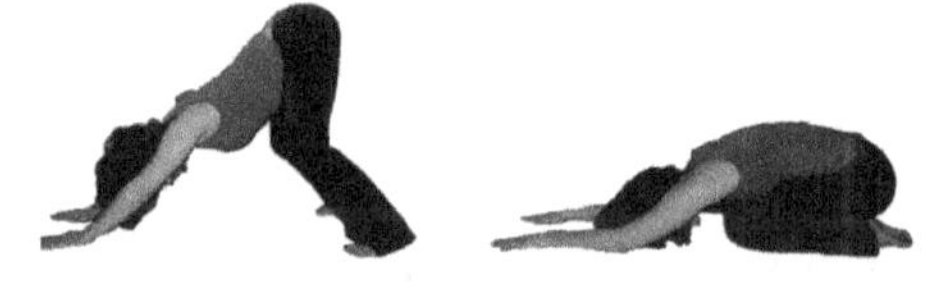

DANDANSA OR STAFF POSE –
5 Breaths
BOAT / FORWARD BEND FLOW –
10 Breaths

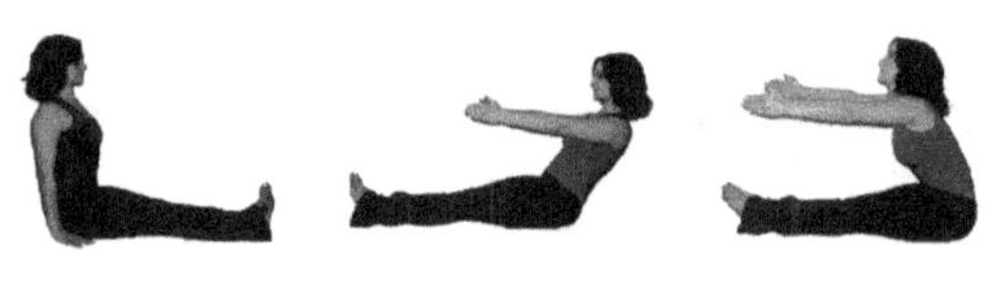

EASY BRIDGE POSE – 5 Breaths
SAVASANA OR RELAXATION POSE
– 10 TO 20 Breaths

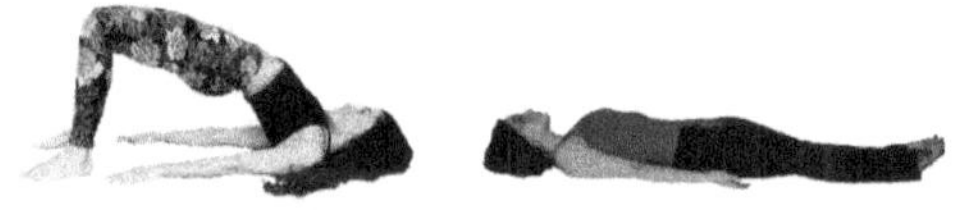

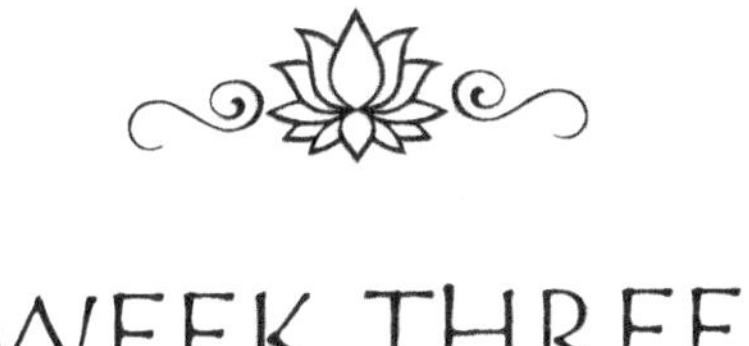

WEEK THREE

INTRO

This week's mind / body vinyasa may be more challenging. For the novice, be gentle by bending the knees when your hands cannot reach the floor. Do what you can do today. Reward yourself for your daily practice with loving thoughts.

DHARMA

Let the ego mind go just for a moment and be content with who you are right now. Release the struggle for perfection and find the joy in the movement, the flow of your breath, the beating of your heart and the rhythm of you.

"Happiness is not something that someone else, like a lover, can give to us. We have to achieve it for ourselves. And the only way to do so is by developing our character and capacity as human beings—by fully maximizing our potential. If we sacrifice our growth and talent for love, we absolutely will not find happiness. True happiness is obtained through fully realizing our potential."
– Daisaku Ikeda

POSTURES (VINYASA)

TADASANA – 5 BREATHS *(WEEK ONE)*

FORWARD BEND FLOW – 10-20 BREATHS *(WEEK ONE)*

CHAIR POSE, *UTKATASANA*

From *Tadasana*, mountain pose, place the feet and knees parallel about hip width distance apart, tilt the sitting bones back and bend the knees as if you are about to sit in a chair. Reach the arms up parallel while relaxing the shoulders down. The palms face inward, and the arms remain shoulder width distance. From here, ground the feet into the earth, stretching up from the sitting bones to the crown of the head and out to the fingers. Now arch the back slightly and lifting the chest. For more advanced students you can clasp the hands above the head for 5-10-breaths.

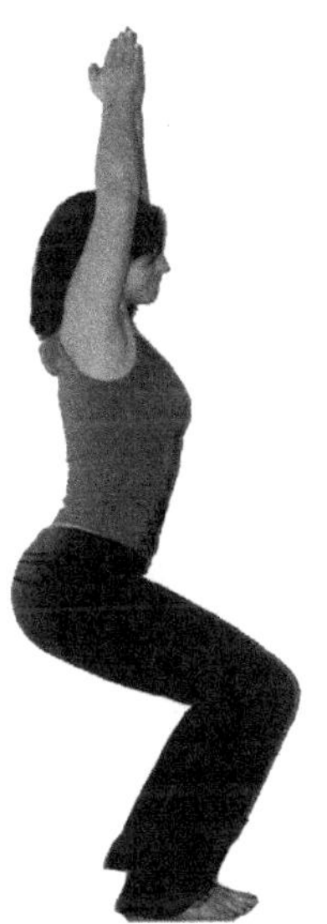

Benefits

Utkatasana strengthens the quadriceps muscles that protect the knees, the hamstring and gluteus muscles, and the muscles in the arms, back and chest. This is also a basic balancing pose that helps to create a more focused mind and balanced life.

WINDMILL POSE

Step the feet about 3-feet apart. The arms extend parallel to the shoulders, reaching out to the sides. Inhale energy, extending from the feet to the crown of the head and out the fingertips (Position A).

Exhale and bend at the hips with the strength of the legs as you drop your left hand to the outside of the right foot. Now twist from the lower, middle to upper back to look up at the right hand. Arms remain parallel (Position B).

You can hold the calf muscle or a block or chair if you cannot reach the foot (Position C).

Powerfully inhale back to the standing posture using the strength of the legs and exhale to the other side. 10-30-breaths

Benefits

This is one of my favorite poses of all times. It's not only fun to do; it's jammed packed with benefits including stretching and strengthening the entire back of the legs and the sides and waist, arms, and neck. It also twists the spine and strengthens the back and sides. It's a great way to focus the mind and invigorate your day if you feel like you're dragging. Try to build up to doing 30 breaths. After you have practiced for a few months and feel confident in this pose, for a real challenge, try doing the magic number - 108.

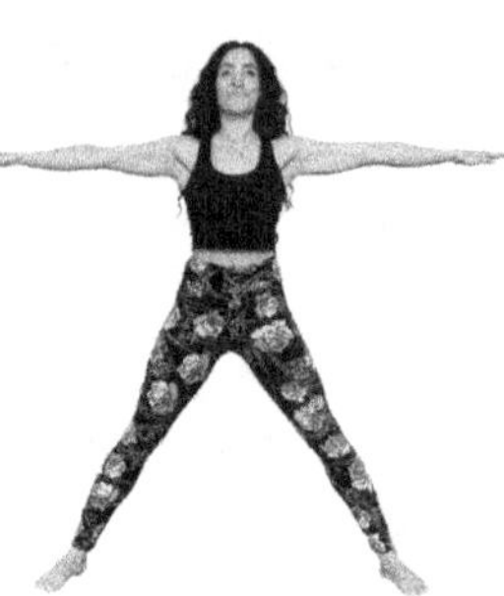

POSITION A

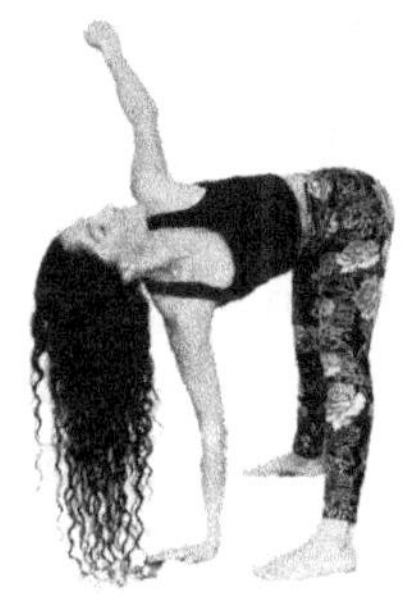

POSITION B

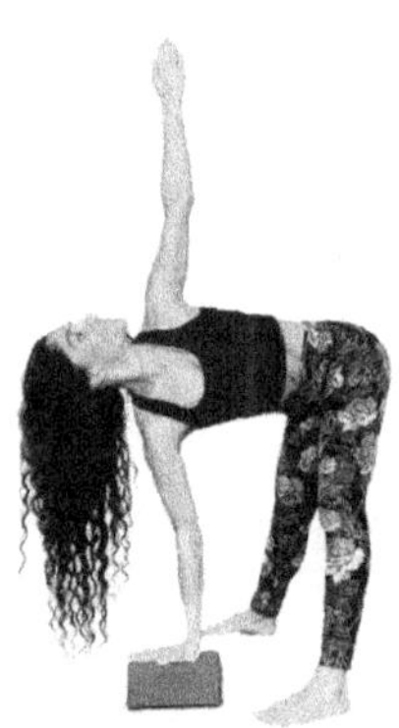

POSITION C

Windmill pose is so easy to do, and you can do it almost anywhere. I often incorporate this pose after a long walk in the park or after a long flight in the airport during a layover. (See Office Ergonomics and Travel)

WINDMILL SIDE STRETCH

Take this pose one step farther with a deeper stretch. On an exhale, bend from the hips, drop both hands down to the floor, placing them under the shoulders (Position A), or place your hands on a block or chair.

Now center your right hand under you and twist, lower, middle, then upper back to look up at your left hand (Position B) for 3-5 breaths.

Return to center (Position A), before preparing the other side.

Benefits

After warming the body and preparing the spine in Windmill flow, Windmill Side Stretch allows you to twist with more control, allowing the breath to release the spine and release deeper into the pose.

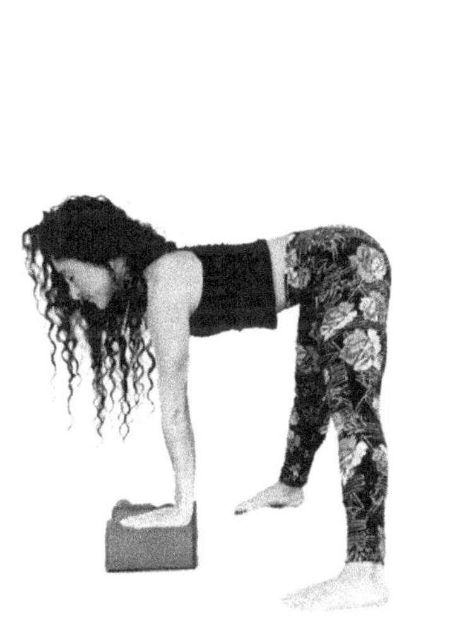

POSITION A

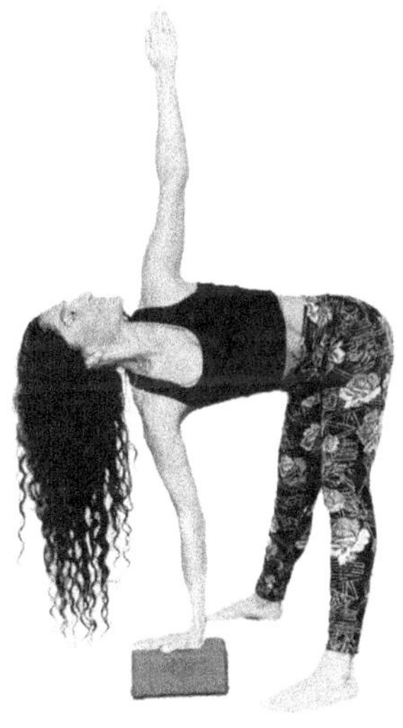

POSITION B

WIDE LEG FORWARD BEND, *PRASARITA PADOTTANASANA*

Place the feet about three feet or more apart and place the hands on the hips. Look up and back and then hinge at the hips while folding forward. Place the hands under the shoulders, look up and stretch the sitting bones up. Try to keep the back arched, not rounded, and take a breath here (Position A).

You may use a block or a chair. Now completely fold forward releasing the head, placing the hands in line with the feet (Position B).

The ultimate goal is to bring the crown of your head down to the floor. Do not force, but allow the breath to release the hips and back deeper into the pose for 5-breaths.

Benefits

This forward bend strengthens and stretches the inner and back legs, and the spine, tones the abdominal organs, calms the brain, and relieves mild backaches.

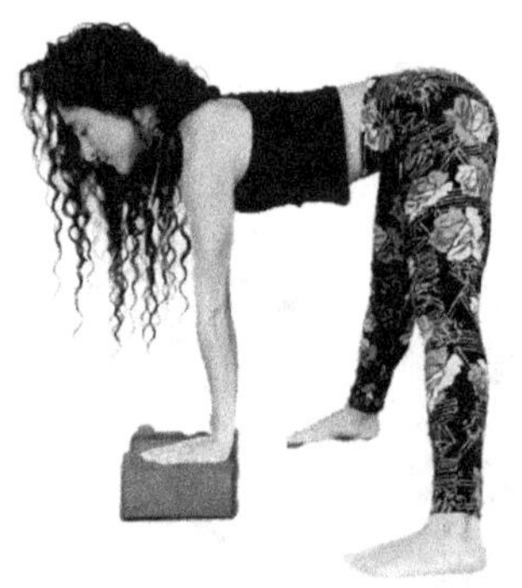

POSITION A

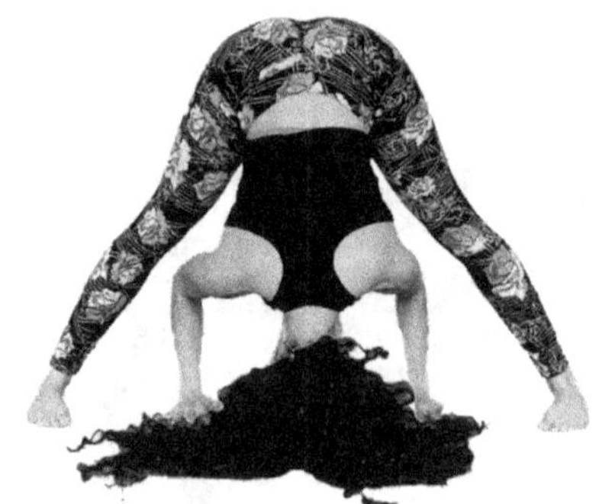

POSITION B

COW-CAT-COW-DOWN DOG FLOW

Now we will combine several poses for an energizing flow. Move to hands under shoulders and knees hip width distance, inhale while lifting the head and sitting bones, letting the spine sink down, arching into Cow Pose.. Then, exhale and tuck the head and sitting bones rounding into cat stretch and inhale again into cow pose.

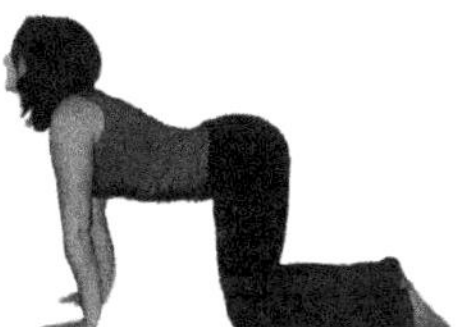

POSITION A

Now, exhale, straighten the legs and push the sitting bones back into down dog, *Adho Mukha Shvanasana*. For the first one, you may try the Bent Knee Forward Bend for a deep stretch and to prepare.

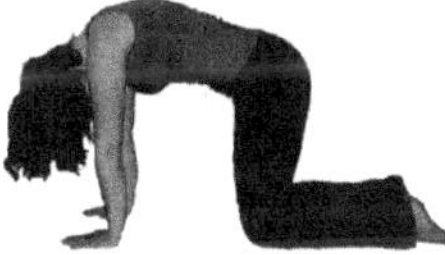

POSITION B

For all others in the series, try with the feet hip width distance apart and the legs as straight as possible. However, the knees remain slightly bent for safety. Never lock the knees in any pose. As you exhale, for a deeper stretch, press the heels down to the floor. Now imagine a string pulling the chest towards to the floor. Hold the first Down Dog for a few breaths then continue the flow.

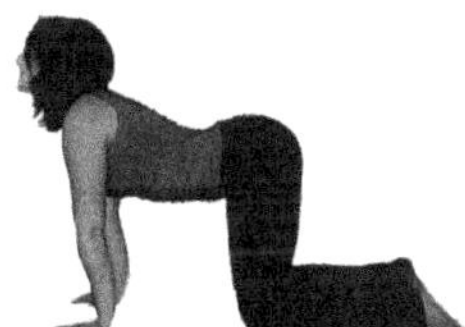

POSITION C

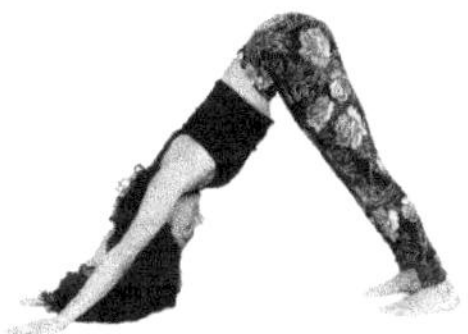

POSITION D

Each pose takes one breath including Down Dog. Flow for at least 10-30-breaths. Let the breath determine the movement.

The most important part of Down Dog is to stretch the spine and hamstrings. If the back is rounded, bend the legs slightly and lift the heels to maintain the stretch in the spine.

Benefits

See Cat / Cow and Down dog. This is one of my favorite flows. It warms and strengthens the entire body and helps to prepare for sun salutations.

DOWN DOG, *ADHO MUKHA SVANASANA*

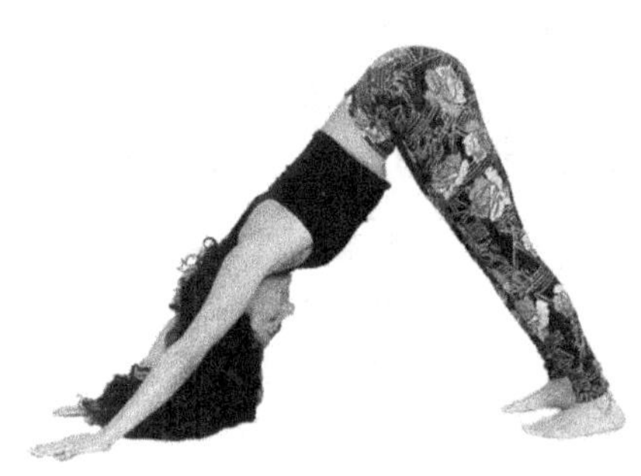

With the fingers spread wide and the index fingers facing slightly outward, push the floor away with your hands. Press the heels down and imagine a string pulling your chest down to the floor while lengthening from the shoulders. As in child's pose the spine lengthens in two directions. The upper back moves down towards the head and the floor, and the sitting bones push back to the ceiling. Relax the neck and head and hold for 5 – 10-breaths.

Benefits

Adho Mukha Svanasana is one of the foundation poses in yoga because it benefits the entire body. It stretches and strengthens the spine, calves, hamstring muscles, ankles, feet, and wrists, relaxes the neck, and promotes tranquility. It's an active and relaxing pose and the center of any good yoga practice.

FALLEN LEAF

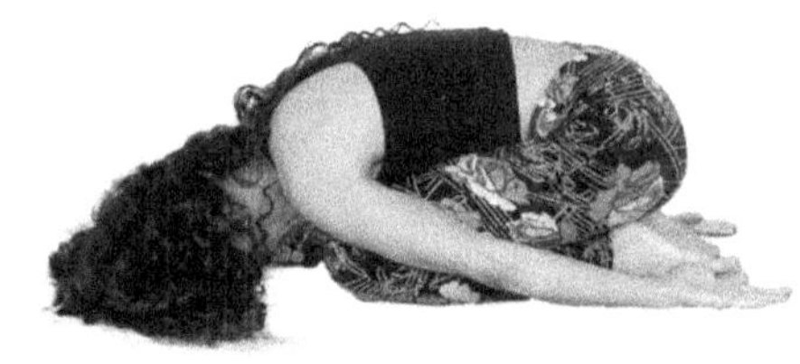

After down-dog, place the sitting bones on the heels, relax the forehead on the mat or a pillow, and wrap the arms around the body with the palms facing up and hands relaxed by the feet. Relax the whole body. Release the shoulders down, allowing the shoulder blades to hang open, and inhale into the lower back for 5-breaths .

Benefits

Fallen Leaf relaxes the shoulders and relieves stress and tension in the lower back. It also gently stretches the quadricep muscles, which help to protect the knees. This is a relaxing pose, great for stress relief.

ONE LEG SEATED FORWARD BEND, *JANU SIRASANA*

From *Dandasana,* Staff Pose with the legs stretched in front of you and the back completely straight. Imagine a string pulling the crown of your head up.

Bend the left leg to place the foot on the inside of the right inner thigh. If you cannot reach the inner thigh comfortably, adjust to above or below the knee.

Now from this position begin to fold forward hinging at the hips to bring your lower belly down to the top of the right leg while you continue stretching the spine upward (Position A).

Make sure you do not round the lower back. If you do, then sit on a pillow. Only bend as far as you can without overstretching the lower back. You should feel this pose mostly in the hamstring muscles.

For more advanced practitioners continue stretching the middle belly, then chest, and relax the head onto a pillow or the legs (Position B) for 5-breaths. Return to *Dandasana* or staff pose then swap sides.

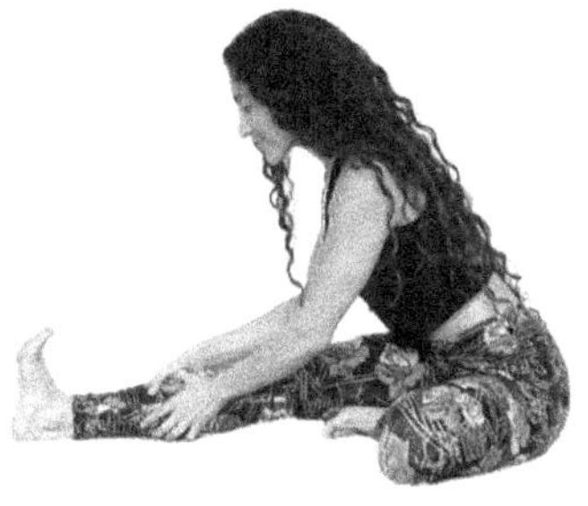

POSITION A

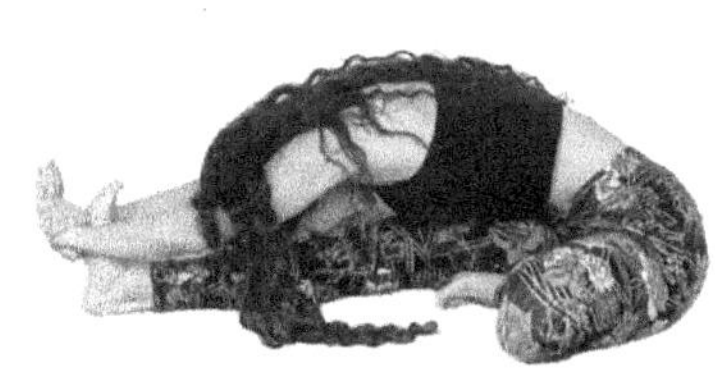

POSITION B

Benefits

Janu Sirasana stretches the spine, hamstring, groins and shoulders, improves digestion, stimulates the liver and kidneys, and relieves anxiety, headaches, and menstrual discomfort. It is also therapeutic for high blood pressure, insomnia, and sinusitis.

EASY BRIDGE – 5 BREATHS *(WEEK TWO)*

CRADLE ROCK

Relax the head and back onto the mat, bring the knees to the chest, and wrap the arms around the legs. Squeeze the legs into the chest and roll side to side on the back for a few wonderful breaths

BENNEFITS

Cradle Rock massages the lower back and is an effective counter pose to all back bending poses.

SAVASANA

By now you know how important this pose is. This week as you relax into your mat, inhale and think *Sat,* pronounced like "but." As you exhale think *Nam,* pronounced like "Mom." These Sanskrit words mean "my true self. " After at least 5-breaths, release the mantra, breathing deeply for a combined total of 10-20-breaths.

A mantra is used to focus the mind and allow it to release ego-based thoughts. Focusing the mind creates a deep feeling of relaxation and peace. You can use this mantra anytime in your day to release tension and improve focus.

HAVE A BLESSED DAY, NAMASTE

Week Three Summary of Poses

TADASANA – 5 Breaths
FORWARD BEND FLOW –
10 Breaths

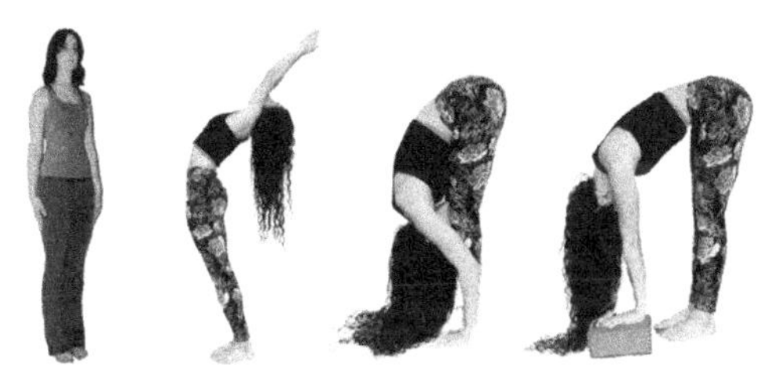

CHAIR POSE UTKATASANA –
5-10 Breaths X 2
WINDMILL – 10 Breaths

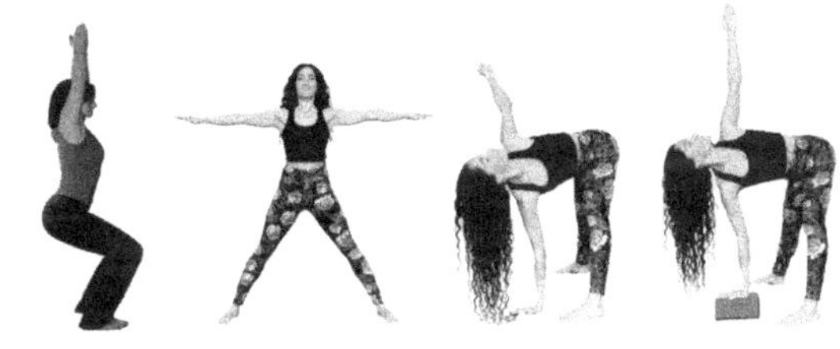

WINDMILL SIDE STRETCH –
3 Breaths X 2
WIDE LEGGED FORWARD BEND –
5 Breaths

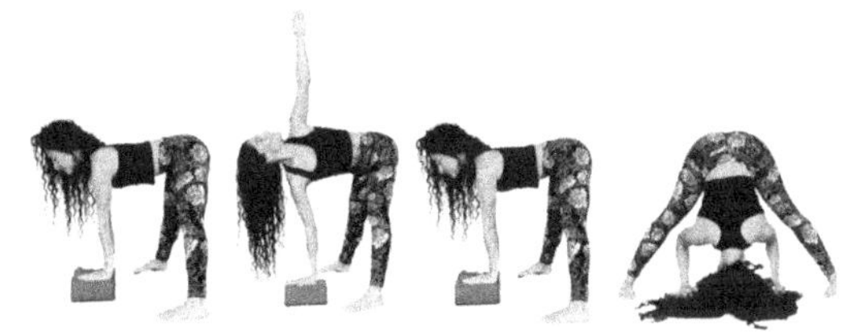

COW-CAT-COW-DOWN DOG
FLOW – 10 Breaths
DOWN DOG – 5 Breaths

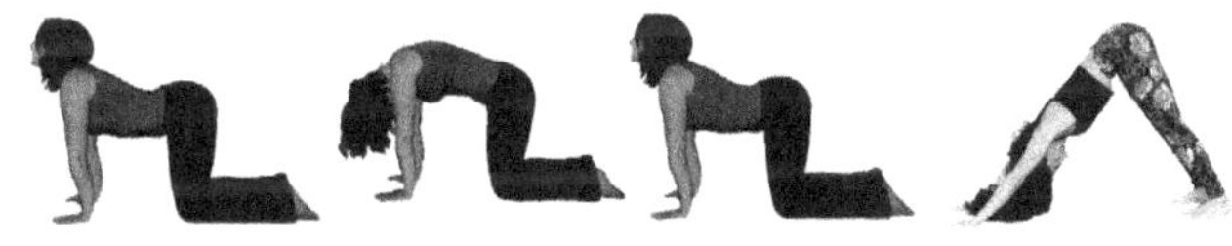

FALLEN LEAF – 5 Breaths
ONE LEG SEATED FORWARD BEND
JANU SIRASANA – 5 Breaths X 2

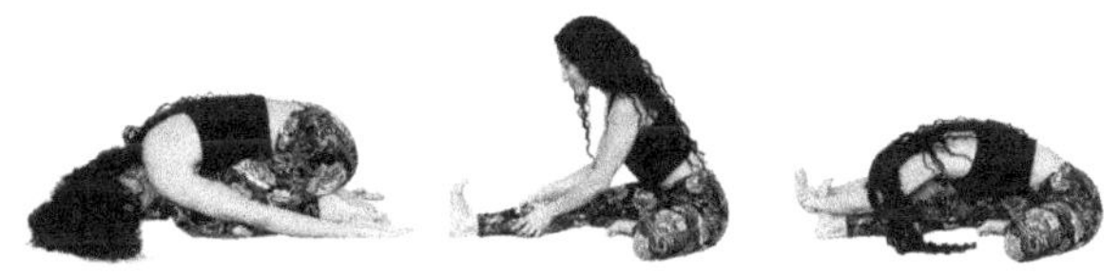

EASY BRIDGE – 5 Breaths
CRADLE ROCK – A few breaths

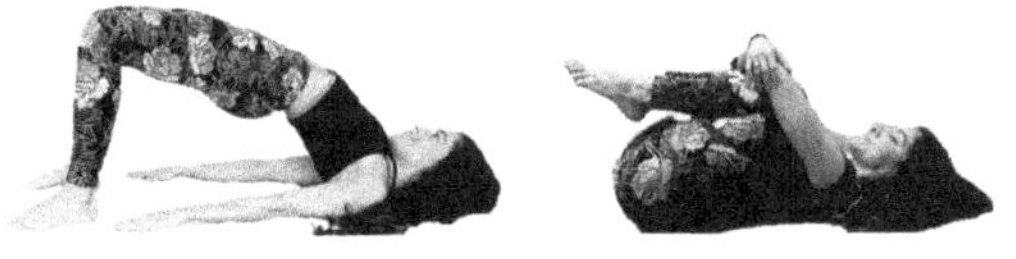

SAVASANA – 10-20 Breaths –
Satnam – 5-10 Breaths –
Release 5 breaths

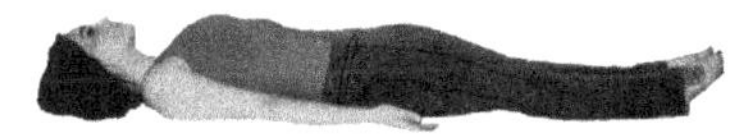

WEEK FOUR

INTRO

This week is especially good for the lower back. I have also included a mild inversion to improve circulation and alleviate the effects of gravity. We continue the poses we've learned and learn to open the lower back, relieving tension by creating more space in the spine and joints. Finally, we conclude with a discussion of control of our thoughts and the effects of this simple practice on our world.

"I alone cannot change the world, but I can cast a stone across the water to create many ripples." – Mother Teresa

DHARMA

Living each day in a way conducive to our higher goals is not easy but can be the most rewarding practice of all. We will not be perfect. We will falter. But at least if we aim to do our best, given our circumstances, we will improve not only our life conditions, but by example and by creating more collective positive energy, the conditions for all of life.

MOUNTAIN POSE, TADASANA – 5-BREATHS *(WEEK ONE)*

TADASANA STRETCH ON TOES

From *Tadasana*, Mountain Pose, inhale the arms above the head to bring the hands together in prayer pose and simultaneously lift the heels rising onto of the toes. While engaging the abdominal / core muscles, stretch the body and spine long as if a string is pulling you up from your fingertips (Position B). As you exhale, lower the arms to the sides and lower the heels down (Position A). Allow the breath to guide this slow and controlled movement. Inhale up and exhale down for 10-breaths.

Benefits

This flow strengthens the ankles and calves, stretches the entire body, and most importantly, develops a sense of balance. With consistent practice you will become more confident in this pose and in life.

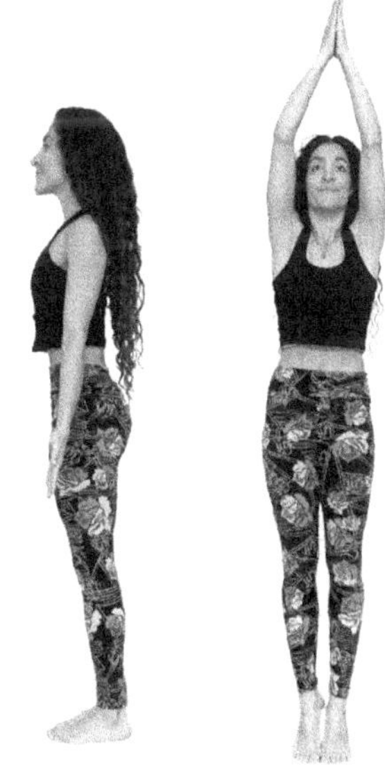

COW-CAT – 5-BREATHS *(WEEK ONE)*

THREAD THE NEEDLE

From Cat / Cow, center the weight over the hands and knees. Twist the torso to gently lift the right arm straight up as you look up and perform a gentle twist from the lower, middle, and upper back. Now slide the right arm under the torso and center the right shoulder. Turn the head to gently look up and stretch the left arm straight up, twisting to left now. The palms face each other. Take 5-breaths on each side.

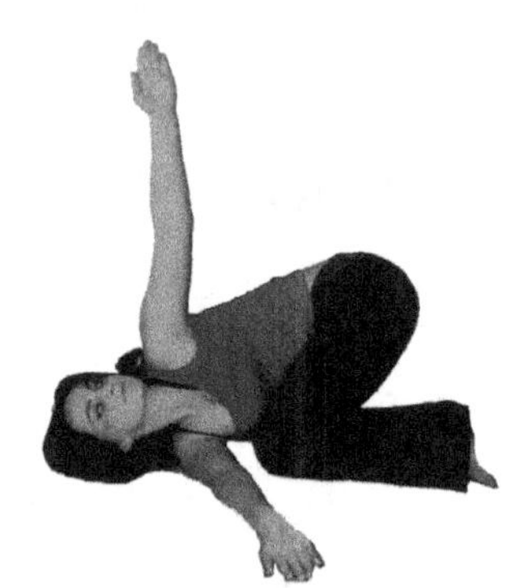

Benefits

This variation of a twist pose safely helps to release the shoulders and assist in twisting the spine and releasing the muscles of the back that can become stuck. Lifting the arm in the beginning is a great chest stretch. Rather than living in a slouched, fearful, unaware posture, when the chest is open and the spine is balanced, we can stand more confident and be more receptive to the possibilities of the world.

As we become stuck in our ways, our spines and the joints become the living evidence of this "stuck-age." The muscles have a memory that communicates with the nerves and the brain. As we do yoga, we are also releasing the past of painful memories and healing wounds that may have been lodged in our muscle memory for decades. This experience can be very cathartic. Do not resist, but let the breath release you. In addition, Twists massage internal organs, which can also hold onto old patterns and outdated ideas. Drink lots of water after all your sessions, just as you would after a massage, so that you can release these old toxic ideas and physical toxins out of your body, mind, and soul.

COW-CAT-COW-DOWNDOG – 10-BREATHS *(WEEK THREE)*

DOWN DOG – 5-BREATHS *(WEEK THREE)*

PLANK, *PHALAKASANA*

From Down Dog come into a push-up position with the hands under the shoulders. Imagine the body as a plank with the abdominal and leg muscles and rotate the elbows to face towards the back body. Open the shoulders by gently pulling them away from the ears, and ground from the hands with the index fingers pointing slightly outward as in down dog. Lengthen from the head to the heels for 5-breaths.

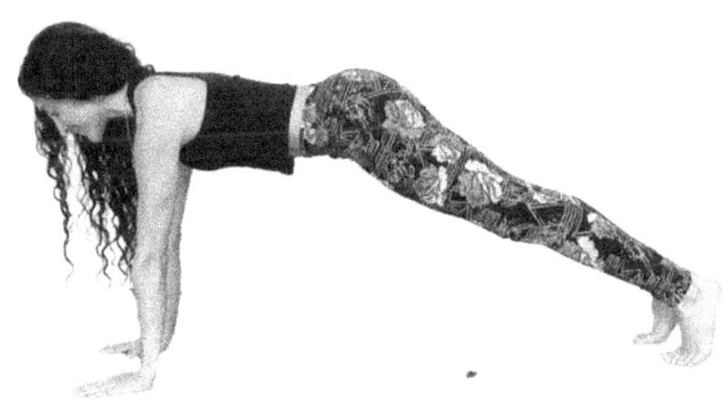

Benefits

Plank Pose strengthens the arms, wrists, and spine, and tones the abdomen. The entire body is toned. This pose develops confidence and strength for future yoga poses and challenges in life.

Plank pose can also strengthen our determination to overcome obstacles that seem to barricade our future progress in our practice and in life. Try doing this pose for longer times like two minutes or up to twenty breaths. Or take brief 2-5 breath breaks and repeat the pose several times for shorter periods. Unlike the traditional push-ups in a gym, *Phalakasana* is a safe way to strengthen the arms, abdominal muscles, and the whole body.

SPHYNX POSE, SALAMBA *BHUJANGASANA*

From Plank, while engaging the abdominal muscles drop the belly down to the mat, letting your chin, chest and knees lead the way. Place the elbows under the shoulders with your forearms resting parallel in front. With hands facing down, spread the fingers wide while lifting the chest like the Egyptian Sphinx. Resist the temptation to crunch the shoulders, but instead open and lengthen by pulling them away from the ears. The legs are extended and parallel to the hips. Make sure to relax the gluteal muscles and point the toes slightly in. Breathe into the lower back for 5-breaths. Continue to lift the chest as you breath and relax the face.

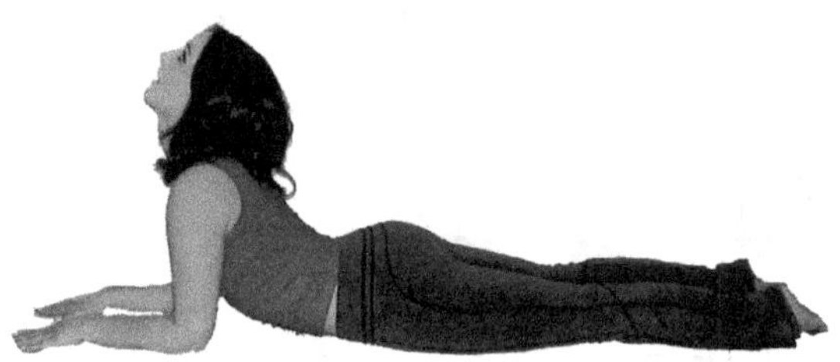

For an additional option between back bending poses, lie on the stomach with the arms by the side and the head turned one way. Relax the spine for 5-breaths. Let the sides relax down to the earth like butter melting to the floor.

Benefits

Sphynx Pose is good for everyone; however, people who sit at desks often, consequently rounding their backs, creating what is known, in ergonomics, as repeated injury to their spines, may especially benefit. While strengthening the back muscles, this pose also helps to put the spine back into its natural posture. It also stretches the chest, shoulders and abdomen, massages abdominal organs and relieves stress in the lower back. Be cautious not to over-extend as this may reverse the benefits of the pose and potentially cause harm.

The best zone for your practice to discover is the one where you are dipping into the challenging edge of postures while staying clear of painful overextending. Your flexibility and stamina will change over time but staying in this zone of challenging comfort is where you will reap the physical, mental, and spiritual rewards of your practice.

Just as Sophocles' Oedipus solved the riddle of the Sphynx to become the leader of Thebes, perhaps we can solve the riddles of our bodies, minds, and souls, to become the leaders of our own lives that we were destined to be.

COBRA FLOW, *BHUJANGASANA*

From Sphynx Pose lie on the belly, place the chin centered on the mat between the hands, which are directly under the shoulders. Try to keep the elbows close to the body and the shoulders away from the ears. The legs are extended with the toes pointed slightly inward. And in all back bending postures practice relaxing the gluteal muscles, which opens the lower back for safely performing back bends. Maintain a bend in the arms as you straighten them a little on the first inhale to arch the chest up and look up. Keep the top of the legs on the mat. Do a little more arching of the back with each breath. The goal is to make a "C" shape with the back. Be mindful not to scrunch the shoulders. Press the shoulders away from the ears as you lift into Cobra Pose. Exhale while bending the arms to return the chin, gently, to the mat. Repeat for 5-breaths, arching and straightening the arms a little more with each inhale.

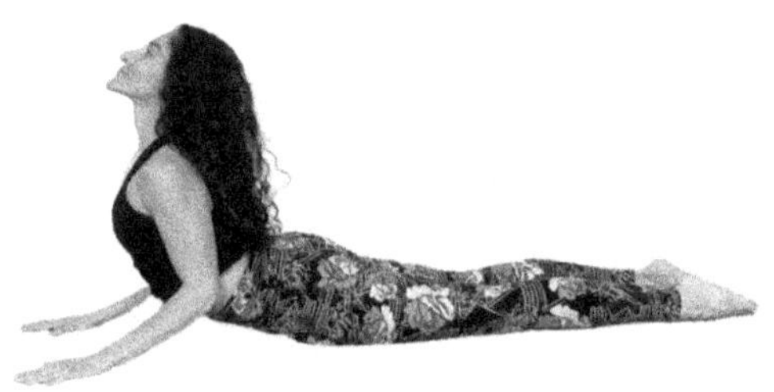

Benefits

According to traditional text, *Bujangasana* increases body heat, destroys disease, and awakens the powerful kundalini energy contained at the base of the spine.

Awakening our kundalini energy can be likened to awakening to our true selves, to the infinite energy we are connected to and part of and ultimately to the awareness that we are one with this universal energy (or God if you choose) and are a composite and representation of the infinite possibilities of this source energy.

KUNDALINI ABDOMINAL STRENGTHENING WITH BREATH OF FIRE

Roll onto the back, stretching the body long. Engage the abdomen while lifting the shoulders and arms a few inches above the mat with the fingers pointing to the toes. Then from the hips, lift the legs so that the feet are a few inches off the ground. For beginners you may keep one foot on the floor doing one leg at a time. Hold the posture and pump the lower belly in breath of fire for 5-10-breaths.

Benefits

This pose strengthens the entire front of the body especially the abdomen, quadriceps, and chest. Most importantly, combined with this healing breath, it detoxifies the organs, stimulates the digestive organs, and helps with elimination. As you progress in your practice, you can relax in between postures and perform this pose three or more times.

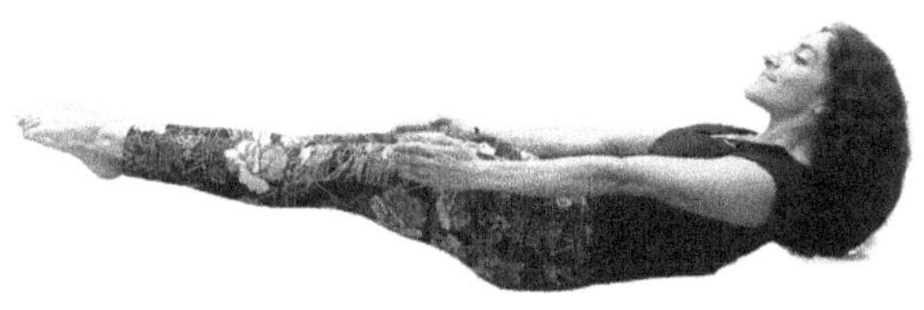

"You surrender to a lot of things which are not worthy of you. I wish you would surrender to your radiance, your integrity, your beautiful human grace." – Yogi Bhajan

MODIFIED SHOULDER STAND, *SALAMBA SARVANGASANA*

Roll the legs and sitting bones up perpendicular to the floor, placing the hands on the hips, keeping the shoulder blades on the floor. The head faces straight with the eyes gazing up at the toes. Imagine a string pulling your toes up to the ceiling (Position A). Make sure the neck is comfortable. There should be no weight on the neck. You may modify to (Position B), halfway up. Take long inhalations and long exhalations for 5-breaths.

Omit this exercise if you have a recent neck injury. You may use an inversion table set at a 45-degree angle for a gentle inversion.

Benefits

Inversion postures reverse the effects of gravity on our bodies by invigorating the skin on the face and neck with fresh oxygenated blood and relieving tension held in the internal organs by reversing gravity. It improves circulation to the heart and the entire circulatory system, which bring oxygen to the entire body. It also drains the lymph system and helps to eliminate fatty deposits in the blood vessels and alleviate varicose veins.

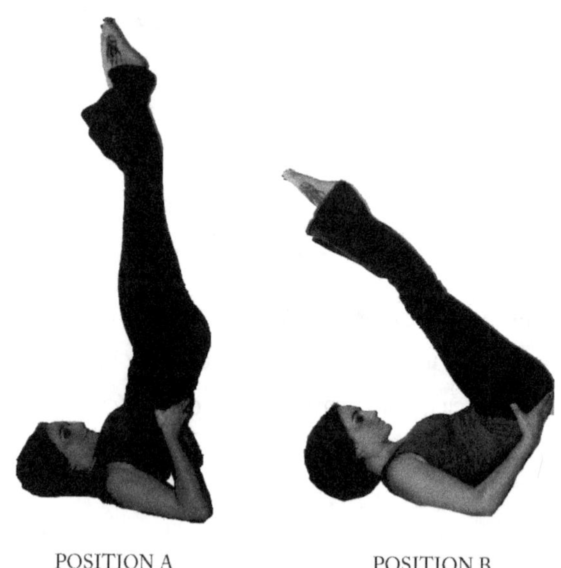

POSITION A   POSITION B

RELAXATION POSE, *SAVASANA*

For this week as you relax onto the mat, breathing through the nose, inhale and think, "Happy am I." Hold the breath as you think, "Healthy am I." Now exhale releasing the breath with, "Holy am I." Remember you are thinking this mantra not speaking it. Completely relax for at least 5-breaths then release the mantra, and enjoy 5 - 30 breaths more as time permits.

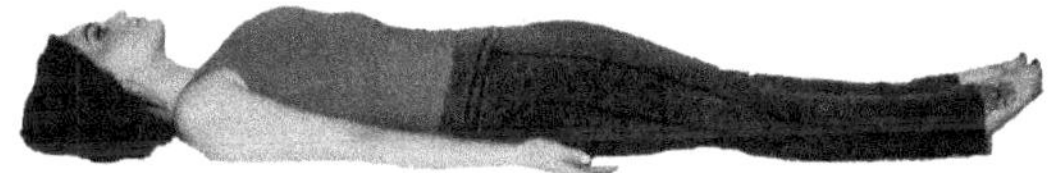

Benefits

This is one of my favorite mantras because it is very simple and yet amazingly effective. You can practice this anytime you are feeling overwhelmed or beginning to get a cold or just need a little pick me up. And you can practice silently anywhere you happen to be.

The benefits of controlling our thoughts are too many to name in this short book. But for the purpose of explaining, I will name a few here. Our thoughts are powerful tools to direct our lives. Contrary to popular belief, we do have control of our minds. It is one of the few things we actually have control over. However, taming this beast is no easy task. And it is not for the weak spirited.

Any attempt to control our "monkey minds" can result in retaliation from our ego, the voice in the head that thinks it is "all that." Once you begin to sit quietly and to plant the seeds of this or another empowering mantra, you may experience some resistance. "This is stupid and a waste of time. We should be working or figuring out what to make for dinner tonight," etc. Just listen to these thoughts as you would listen to a child. Listen patiently, but do not give in to these whims or take them too seriously.

You will find in a short time that you feel more relaxed in general and will become less affected by external circumstances. An irate shopper may cause you to feel compassion for someone who is suffering, rather than outrage. You will begin to inflict less violence against yourself via your words and thoughts and therefore, against others. As we shine the light of awareness on our thoughts and choose empowering thoughts over negative ones, we will likely begin to become kinder and gentler to, not only others, but to ourselves.

When humans take control of their thoughts, and stop the violence in their heads, there is hope that we may then evolve to become a more peaceful species. And since we are all connected via the threads of life that bind us, by practicing yoga you will begin to create a more peaceful world by beginning to create that world every day on the mat with yourself. And once more and more people take up the challenge of controlling the mind, when a critical mass has been reached, all humans will make the leap into living in harmony with themselves and all others.

If everyone demanded peace instead of another TV set,
then there'd be peace.
– John Lennon

HAVE A BLESSED DAY, NAMASTE

Week Four Summary of Poses

TADASANA – 5 Breaths
STRETCH ON TOES –
10 Breaths

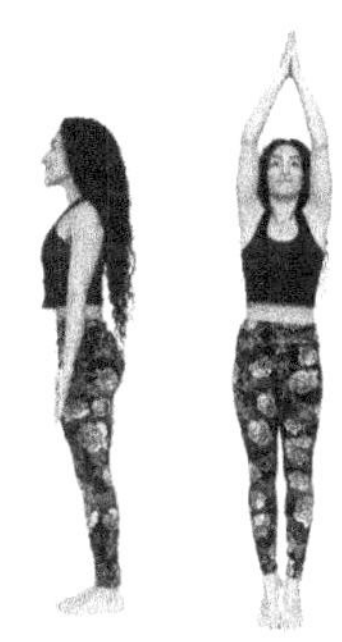

COW-CAT – 5 Breaths
THREAD THE KNEEDLE – 5 Breaths
X2

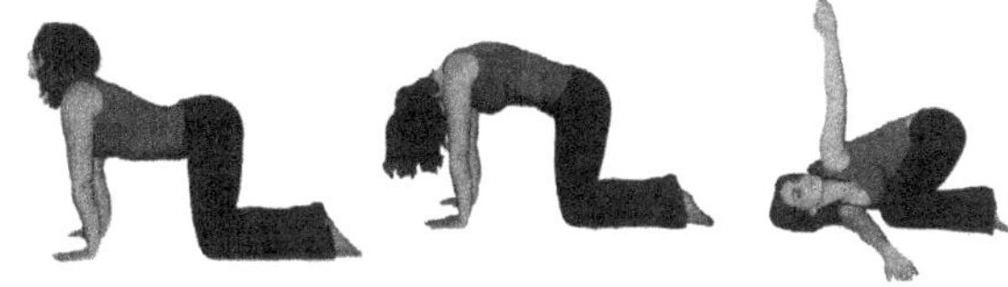

COW-CAT-COW-DOWNDOG –
10 Breaths
DOWN DOG – 5 Breaths

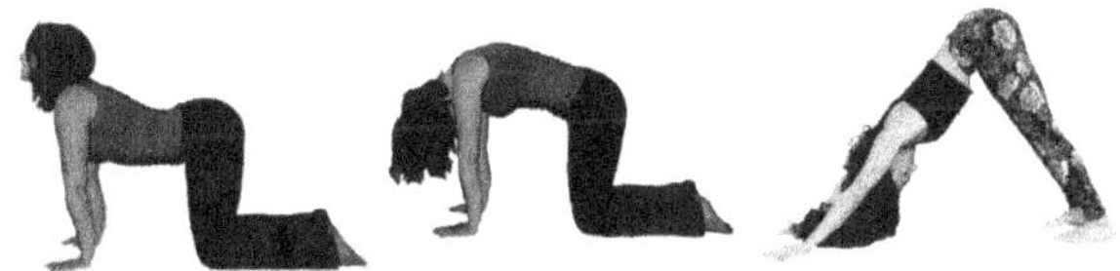

PLANK – 5 Breaths
SPINX – 5 Breaths

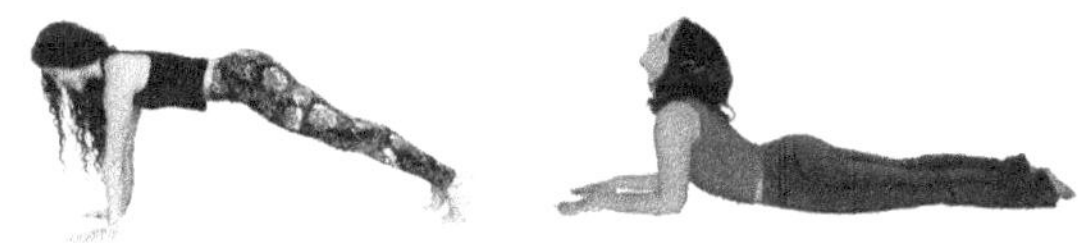

COBRA FLOW – 5 Breaths
KUNDALINI ABDOMINAL WITH
BREATH OF FIRE – 5-10 Breaths

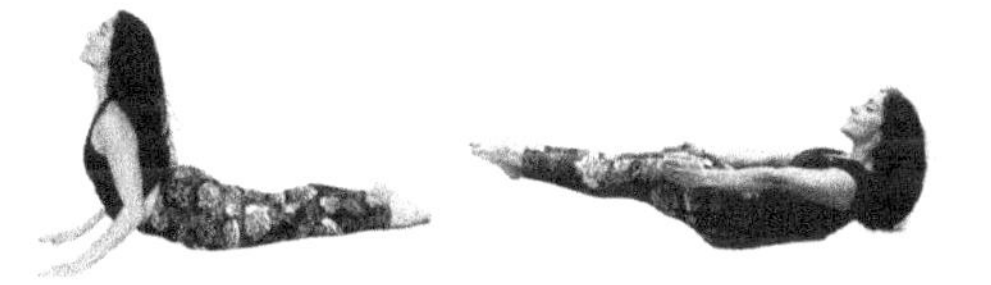

MODIFIED SHOULDER STAND – 5
Breaths
SAVASANA - HAPPY - HEALTHY -
HOLY – 5 Breaths **- RELEASE**

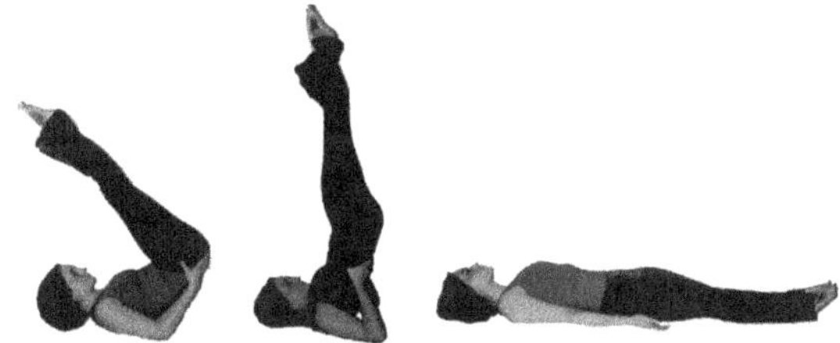

WEEK FIVE

INTRO

Today you are ready to salute the sun as the ancients did long ago. Practice Proud Warrior Pose for the spiritual warrior within and Upward Bow Pose to challenge you to open your heart more than you thought was possible.

DHARMA

We can all live in grace and love. We can all be our true divine expressions. When we realize that we are more than the wave that we ride upon and exist as, and that what lies inside of us is infinitely vast, and that what lies inside and around all other waves is the same vastness, as a species we may experience compassionate peace as never before. Every day is a day to begin again to transform ourselves. We become what we perceive; yet we are always the depth behind the image.

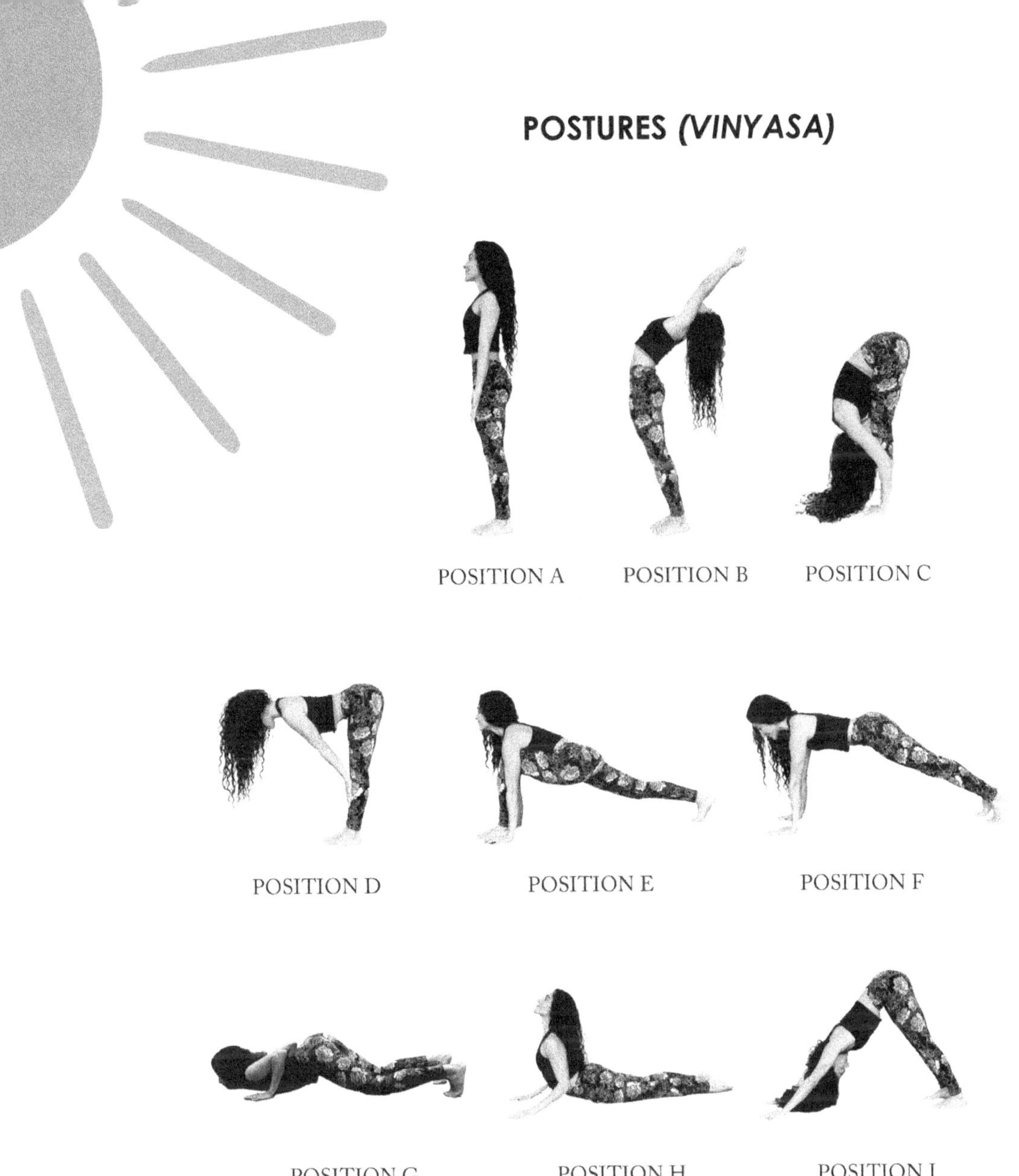

4 SUNSALUTATIONS, *SURYA NAMASKARA*

Begin in *Tadasana* (Position A) Mountain Pose. Then inhale the arms above the head, stretching up and back, bringing the hands together in prayer (Position B). Exhale and stretch the arms along the sides. Hinging at the hips, fold forward, drop the head, and bring the hands to the floor, block or chair. Release the back in *Paschimottanasana*, Standing

Forward Bend, (Position C). Inhale hands on the shin to look up to stretch and straighten the spine, Halfway Up Pose (Position D).

LUNGE POSE, ANJANEYASANA

Now step the right leg back to Lunge Pose, (Position E) *Anjaneyasana*, keeping the left foot under the left knee, and the right leg straight but not locked with the right foot flexed, resting the weight on the toes and ball of the foot. Place the fingertips or hands on yoga blocks or on the ground beside you. Lift the chest; deepen in the stretch by dropping down into the lung a little more. Breathing deeply, 2-breaths.

Benefits

Lunge pose stretches the groin muscles and the entire length of the legs, creates balance and strength and relieves sciatica pain.

CONTINUE THE SUN SALUTATIONS

Place your left foot back to Plank Pose, (Position F), hold for 2-breaths.

Exhale knees, chest, and chin down to the mat (Position G). Inhale lift the heart forward into Cobra Pose to look up at the ceiling (Position H).

Exhale come down to the mat and push back to Downward Facing Dog Pose (Position I). Hold for 2 breaths.

Now bring the right foot forward between the hands for Lunge Pose on the other side (Position E). Hold for 2 breaths.

Bring the left foot forward, place the hands on the shins and look up stretching the spine in Halfway Pose (Position D). Exhale fold forward to a Standing Forward Bend (Position C), lifting the sitting bones, and release for 2 or more breaths.

Hinging at the hips, inhale with the strength of the legs to look up and back (Position B). Exhale the hands in prayer pose in front of your heart.

Now begin again, two sequences beginning with the right leg back and two with the left leg back first. Repeat, as time permits. For a heart invigorating, detoxifying, aerobic experience you may perform 10 - 20 times. This is not part of your ten-minute daily ritual unless you want to extend your time. But this extended series could be added to a weekly ritual.

Benefits

Surya Namaskara, Sun Salutation, tones organs, strengthens the abdominal muscles, ventilates the lungs, oxygenates the blood, detoxifies the body, refreshes the skin, reduces fat, improves muscle flexibility, reduces stress held in the body and mind, and enhances youthful vigor. This is a powerful, mother of all yoga, amazing sequence of poses that almost anyone can do.

TREE POSE, *VRIKSHASANA*

From *Tadasana* or Mountain Pose, shift the weight onto the right foot. Now lift the left foot and place it either with the toes resting on the floor (Position A), against the right heal or on the inside of the right calf (Position B), or on the inner right thigh (Position C). Press the foot firmly into the thigh. Keep your right leg strong, but do not lock the knees. Place your hands in prayer in front of your heart. Gaze at a spot in front of you to remain balanced. Lift the chest. Imagine a string of energy pulling you up from your right foot to the crown of your head. Gently tuck the tailbone and stretch the crown of the head up. For a more advanced hand position, place the hands in prayer straight up above the head and imagine energy pulling them up (Position D). Hold for 5-breaths. This pose may take some practice to achieve and hold. If you have to regain your balance by placing the foot down, just begin again without judgment. Do not worry about beginning with your toes slightly touching the floor; this is a very good place to begin.

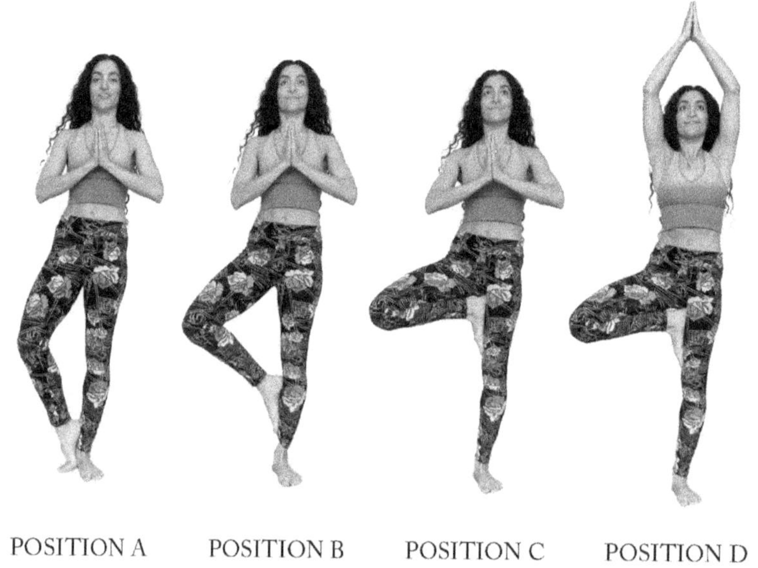

POSITION A   POSITION B   POSITION C   POSITION D

Benefits

This pose focuses the mind, creates more balance in the body, and strengthens the feet, ankles, spine, legs and groin.

SIDE STRETCH, *PARSVAKONASANA*

Step the feet about 3 or more feet apart, turning the right foot perpendicular to the left, and bend the right knee over the right foot. Lift the arches of the left foot, place the right forearm over the right quadriceps and stretch the left arm parallel with the torso over the head. The hips are facing forward (Position A). After practicing many times or if you are more flexible, you may place the right hand next to the foot (Position B). Gaze straight ahead, at the ceiling, or at the fingers of the left hand, which ever feels comfortable on your neck, and open the chest up to the sky for 5-breaths. If you feel unnecessary tension in the neck, continue to gaze forward. Inhale and with the strength of both legs return to center and prepare the other side.

Benefits

Strengthens abdominal organs, tones liver and spleen, improves digestion, strengthens, and stretches the legs, hips, and torso, calms the mind, and sooths the nerves.

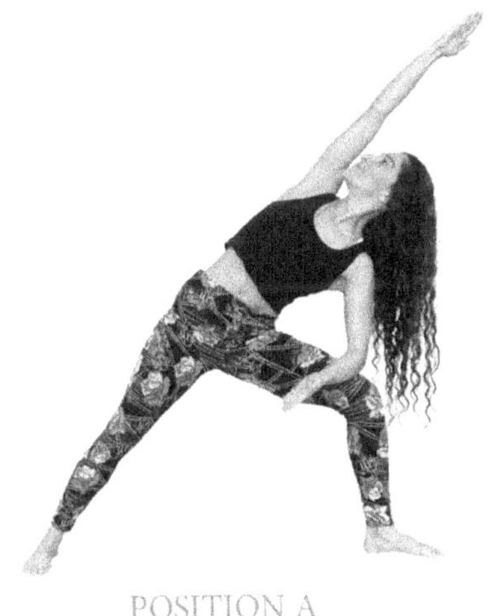

POSITION A

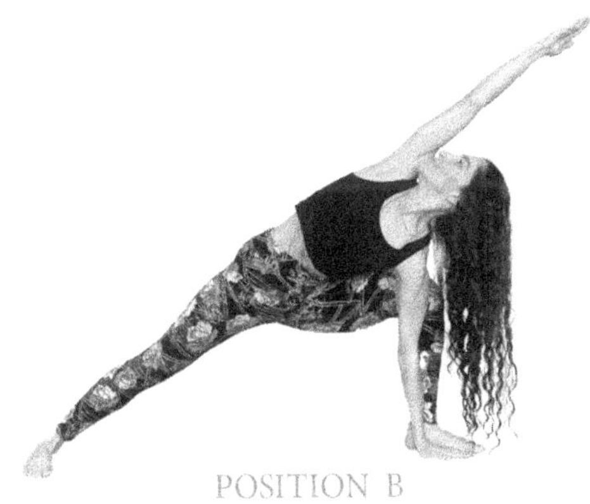

POSITION B

WARRIER II POSE, *VIRABHADRASANA II*

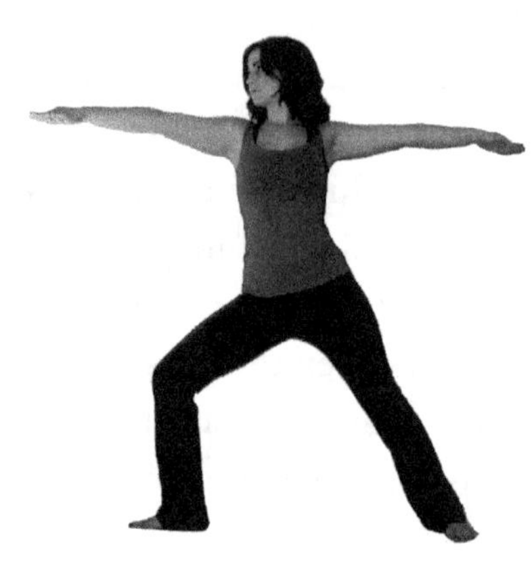

Begin with the feet about 3 or more feet apart. Ground the feet and lift the arches. Lift the chest, turn the right foot 90 degrees, and bend the right knee over the right foot. For the safety of the knee, keep the bent knee in line with the foot. The torso should remain facing in the same direction as the left foot, forward. Place the arms straight out to the sides parallel the torso and the shoulders. Gently press the shoulders down and imagine energy flowing from your feet to your fingertips, stretching in all directions. Now turn and gaze over your right arm for 5-breaths. Inhale back to center and prepare the other side.

Benefits

Named after the warrior Shiva, this pose stretches the groin, chest, and shoulders, stimulates abdominal organs, and increases stamina, strengthens the legs, opens the hips and chest, and develops concentration and grounded-ness. It also strengthens the arms and shoulders.

MINI SUN SALUTE

Return to a lunge position and place the hands on the floor parallel with the forward foot. Step the forward foot back to Plank Pose and exhale down to the mat, leading with the knees, chest, and chin.

BOW POSE, *DHANURASANA*

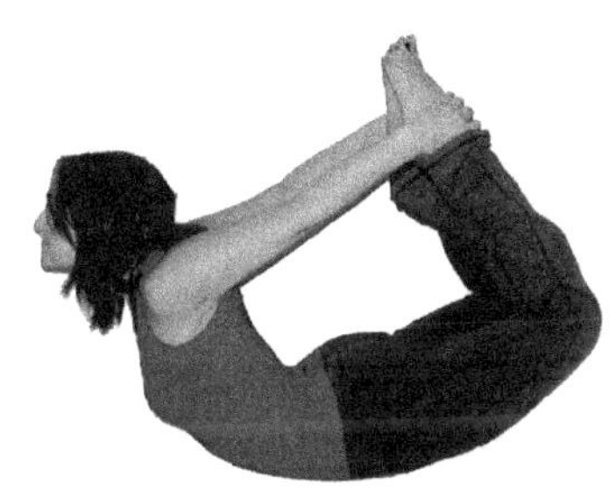

Lying face down, take your right hand to hold the right ankle. If you cannot reach the ankle, you may use a strap or tie. Then take the left hand to hold the left ankle and inhale the chest and legs up as high as you can for 5-breaths. You may roll back and forth as you breath; this is normal. You can do one leg at a time if you are just beginning or have some difficulty holding both ankles.

Benefits

Bow Pose increases strength and flexibility along the entire length of the spine. It lengthens the spine, stretches the neck, shoulders, arms and legs, massages internal organs, and improves digestion. It also helps regulate the pancreas and is recommended for people with diabetes. By reversing irregular curvatures of the spine, it helps alleviate the hunchback condition many office workers develop from slouching in chairs. As the spine is aligned, circulation and concentration improve.

EXTENDED CHILD'S POSE – 5 BREATHS *(WEEK ONE)*

SEATED FORWARD BEND, *PASCHIMOTTANASANA*

Begin in Dandasana (Position A), lift from the sitting bones to the crown of the head, and stretch from the hips to the heels; then hinging at the hips, begin to fold forward. Try to keep the lower back from rounding by releasing the lower belly to the upper thigh first, then the middle belly, then the chest, and relax the head on the legs. I tell my students to imagine that they are releasing even if they are not yet able to fold forward. Most people will make a 45-degree angle with the legs and torso (Position A) before achieving (Position B). Be present with wherever you are in the pose without judgement. Release for 5-breaths.

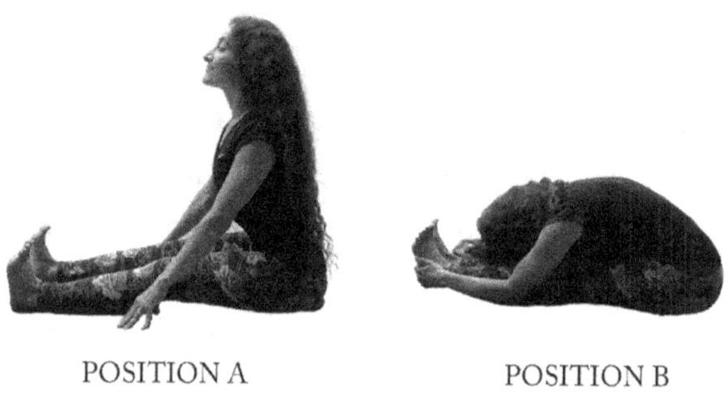

POSITION A   POSITION B

Be aware not to over stretch the lower back as this would be counterproductive to your practice and could be harmful. Let the lower back release, while keeping the hinge of movement focused at the hip area. Resist the temptation to round the back but continue to stretch the spine long.

Benefits

The entire nervous system is invigorated by doing this pose because all the connecting nerves that run along the back of the legs are invigorated by stretching the hamstring, calf, ankle, and foot muscles. It allows the lower back muscles to stretch and release tension. Stretching the leg muscles that connect to the lower back muscles also helps to protect the lower back from injury.

BOAT POSE, *PARPURNA NAVASANA*

You may revert to modified boat pose at this time (Position A). But if you feel limber and strong enough, I encourage you to continue the challenge. From Dandasana, Staff Pose, bend the knees and place the palms next to the knees. Shift the weight back to lift the legs from the hips off the ground. Now only if you feel strong in your core and are flexible enough, straighten the legs to make a 45-degree angle with the body and legs. Hands hover parallel with the knees. Gaze up at the toes, breathing deeply for 5-breaths (Position B). Relax for a moment by pulling the knees into the chest from a sitting position and repeat. Three or more times is ideal.

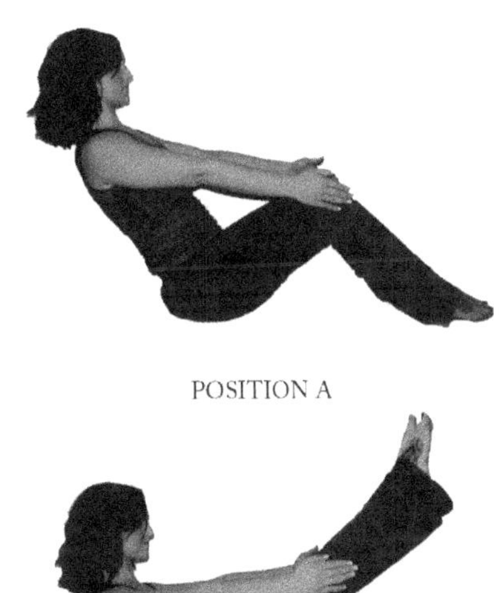

POSITION A

POSITION B

SAVASANA

Lying flat on your mat, release the body a little more with each exhale. Imagine inhaling peace and harmony and exhaling peace and harmony for 10 - 20 beautiful breaths.

HAVE A BLESSED DAY, NAMASTE

Week Five Summary of Poses

---

3 SUNSALUTATIONS

SIDE STRETCH – 5 Breaths X 2
WARRIER POSE – 5 Breaths X 2

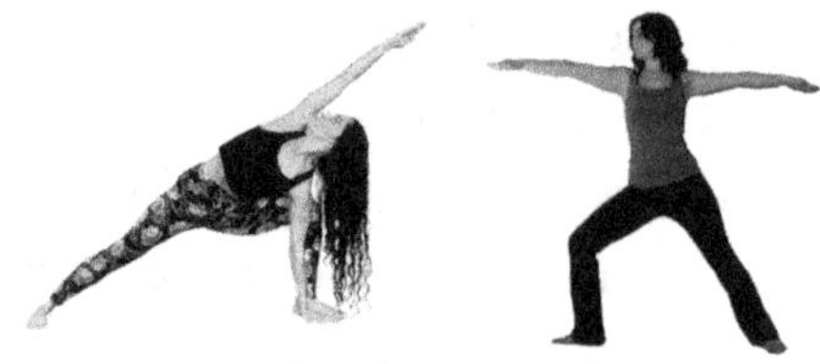

MINI SUN SALUTE
UPWARD BOW – 5 Breaths

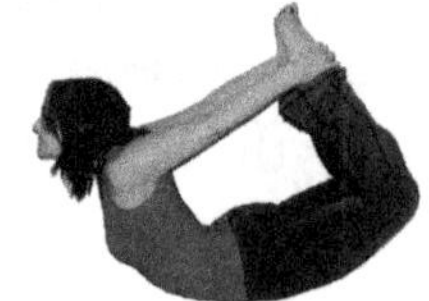

EXTENDED CHILD'S POSE –
5 Breaths

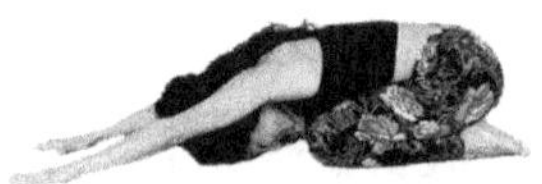

SEATED FORWARD BEND –
5 Breaths
BOAT POSE – 5 Breaths X 2

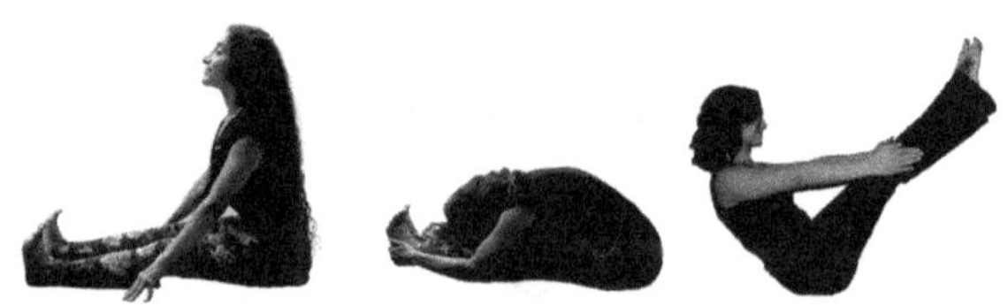

SAVASANA - 10 TO 20 Breaths
RELEASE

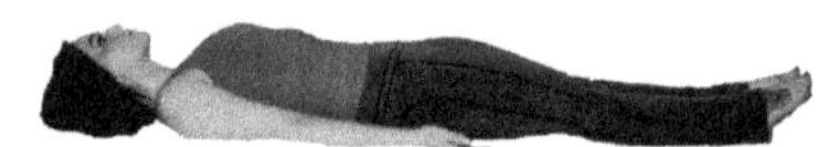

WEEK SIX

INTRO

The Five Tibetans, by Christopher S. Kilham, is a book of a series of postures derived from the Tibetan monks. It is the practice that many monks perform daily as part of their spiritual asceticism and is so amazingly simple and effective that almost anyone can do them with ease and at the same time achieve great results. My friend's sixty-year-old father began practicing these simple poses that take only ten minutes per day and was able to lose fifty pounds in three months. From the moment he began this practice, he said he immediately felt more energized.

DHARMA

Beginning any new activity is the hard part. But continuing after the going gets tough or the going gets much easier is also the hard part. When we begin to feel better and more like ourselves, we may be tempted to stop the process of healing since we have temporarily achieved an intended goal. We may also feel great and become engaged in more activities, which takes our mental, physical and spiritual energy and takes time away from our practice.

The goal of yoga is not to live on the mat, but rather, to take the inner peace, that is created through the practice, out into the *Maya* or material world. However, friends may notice a shift in our energy and subconsciously want to pull us away from our healing journeys as our well-intended friends and family may feel us pulling away from them. Rather than let them do that, we can help others to achieve their goals by sharing our experiences and successes with them. By being living examples of over-coming obstacles and challenges, we are feeding others the necessary hope to achieve their own successes.

If by now, you are practicing more than 10-minutes per day, great. But if you do not have the time for three sessions or for longer sessions, don't deny yourself the 10-minutes of sacred pleasure you deserve.

And by this time, you may be physically able to perform the total 21 times per Tibetan Rite posture, rather than the 10 suggested below. However, to thoroughly experience these postures for the first time, I have suggested starting with 10 and then building to the full 21.

CLOCKWISE SPINS

Stand with the feet a little more than hip distance apart with the arms straight out to the sides parallel with the shoulders. Now begin to spin, but keep the eyes gazing straight ahead. Do not turn the head as dancers do to keep the eyes from spinning. You want to feel the spinning. Spin 10 times.

Benefits

Spinning has been used by sages, like the whirling Dervishes, for centuries. It also balances the right and left energy of the body known as *Nadis* and helps with equilibrium and, with consistent practice, can reduce symptoms of seasickness.

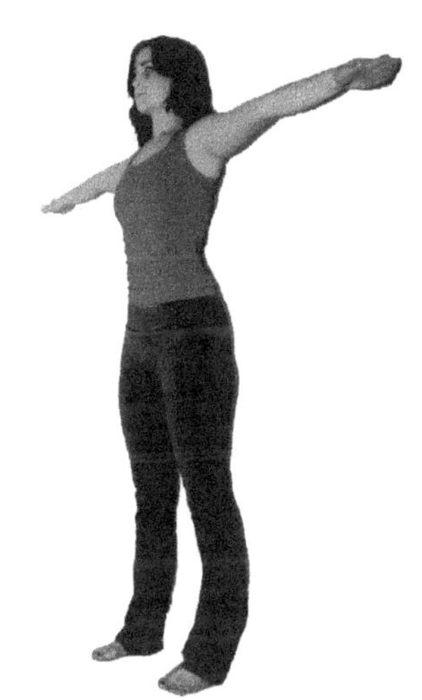

WHISPER BREATHS

When you have finished, perform 3-Whisper Breaths by placing the hands on the hips, inhaling through the nose, exhaling through the whisper lips for 3 breaths. If you need a few more to regain balance, just take them.

Benefits

Whisper Breathing creates sounds that help to focus the mind, but they are also said to help detoxify the body and calm the nervous system.

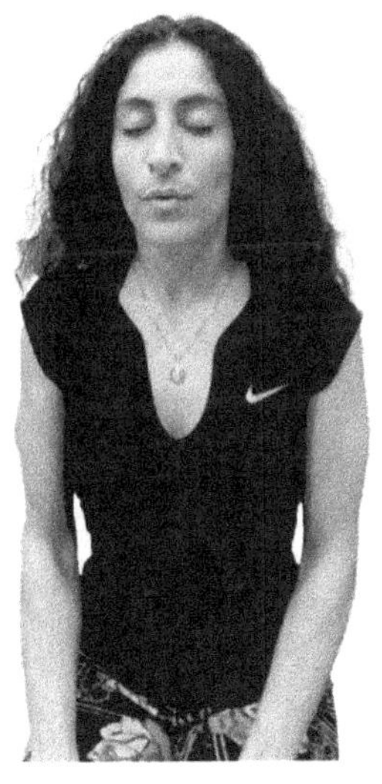

ABDOMINAL LEG LIFTS

Lie on the floor with the palms, facing down, placed under the sides of the sitting bones to protect the lower back. Inhale and lift the legs perpendicular to the floor while lifting the shoulders and slightly tucking the chin. Exhale, release the pose returning the heels to the floor. Keep the shoulders lifted for 10-breaths.

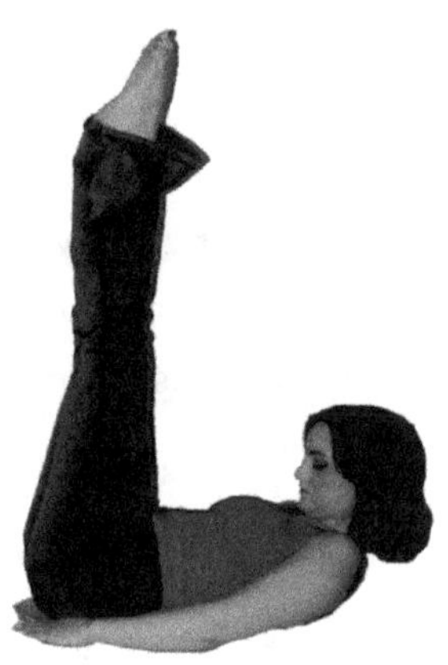

If you feel stress or tension in the neck, you can return your head and shoulders to the floor to relax while you lift the legs in the pose.

When you are finished, roll up to standing and enjoy 3-Whisper Breaths.

Benefits

Leg lifts strengthens the entire front of the body, especially the abdominal area. The strong abdominal muscles not only protect the spine and back muscles from injury, but they also help to center and ground us so that we may make more powerful decisions for ourselves, those we love, and ultimately for the world.

The chakras are energy centers that correspond to points on the spine and the body and are represented by colors. The abdominal area is called the Solar Plexus Chakra. It is yellow like the sun. We can think of this powerful glowing center of our body like the center of our galaxy, our sun, which radiates, not just light, but hope and life itself. Without it, we would not exist. Perhaps keeping our center strong is as important for our bodies as the sun is to our Earth.

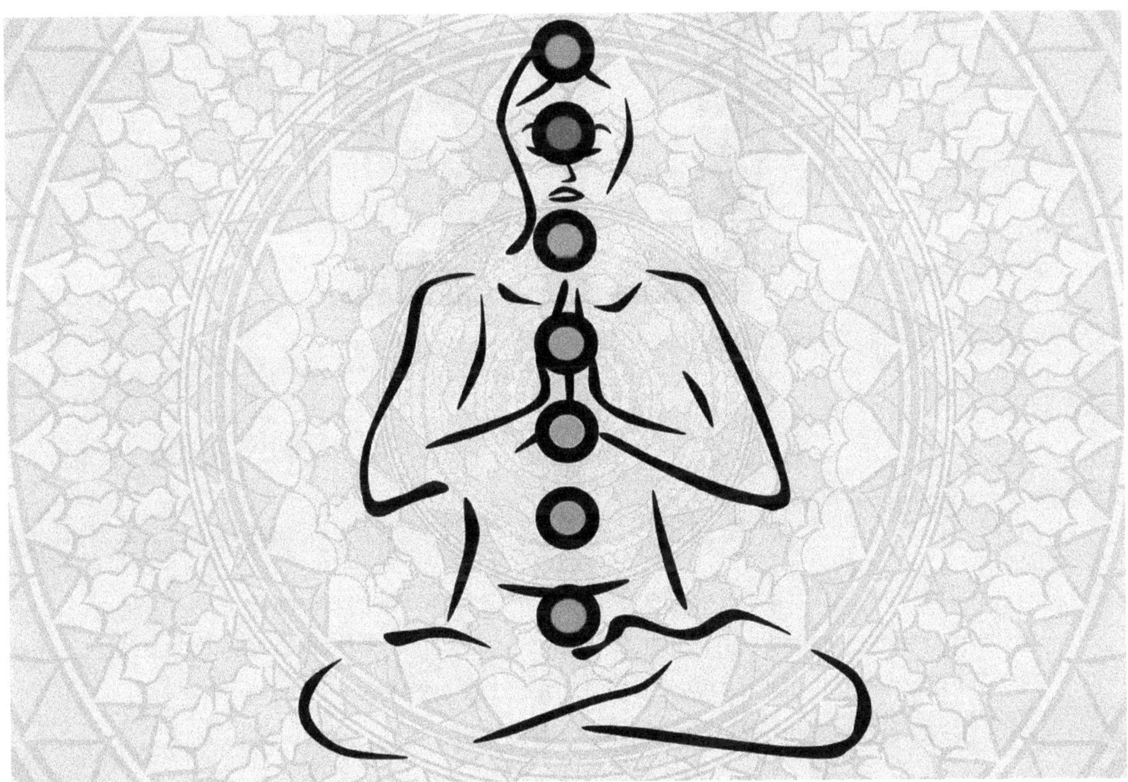

CAMEL FLOW POSE

Begin on the knees and balls of the feet with the hands placed under the sitting bones. Slightly tuck the chin and imagine energy flowing up through the crown of the head (Position A). Inhale and begin to arch back, starting with the head, making a backwards "C" with the spine (Position B). Exhale, return to neutral and slightly tuck the chin. When you have completed 10-breaths, stand, and perform 3-Whisper Breaths.

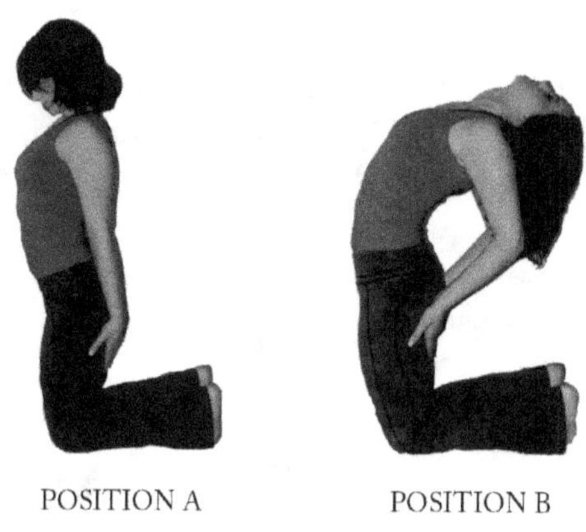

POSITION A   POSITION B

After a neck injury, while performing Camel Pose Flow, my neck would sometimes flop backwards, often over stretching. If you have neck issues, be gentle. You can try using a supportive travel pillow that wraps around the neck and helps to support the neck as you continue to open the chest and stretch in the pose. Eventually, you will build the neck muscles and be able to take the pillow away as I have done.

Also, feeling lightheaded may be a normal response
to newly practicing back bending and chest opening
postures. Return to deep breathing, and this feeling should
subside in a few breaths.

Benefits

Camel Flow stretches the front of the body, arches the spine, and moves the joints. Like all back bending poses, it opens the chest and helps to counter the effects of sitting for long periods or unnatural rounding of the back. The spine was designed to be moved in all directions. Unfortunately, in our society, adults seldom move their spines naturally as children do. So doing back bending poses like camel pose or camel flow will help to counter the effects of stagnation. Movement of the spine oils the joints and keeps them healthy. Camel flow is a safe, invigorating backbend flow.

STAFF TO BRIDGE POSE

Begin in *Dandasana*, Staff Pose, slightly tuck the chin, flex the feet, ground the legs, with the arms by the side and fingers pointing forward (Position A). Inhale lift the sitting bones and torso up and drop the head back to be parallel with the torso. To protect the knees, try to keep them over the feet with the toes facing forward, (Position B). The pose looks like a tabletop. Exhale return to *Dandasana*. On completion of 10-breaths, return to standing for 3-Whisper Breaths.

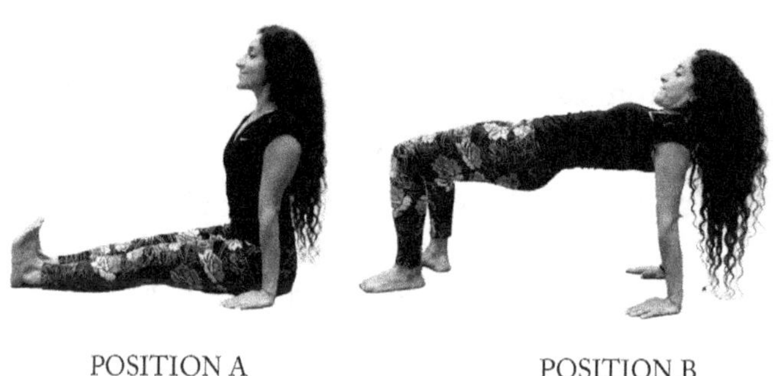

POSITION A   POSITION B

Benefits

Bridge Pose strengthens the quadriceps muscles, arms, shoulders, back and abdominal muscles. It is also helpful in building the strength and endurance necessary for performing more advanced back bending postures.

What is true victory in life? What is the meaning of true happiness? Who is truly great? The answer to such questions is determined not by superficial criteria such as fame, status and wealth, but by the inner reality of one's heart. - Daisaka Ikeda

UPWARD FACING DOG / DOWNWARD FACING DOG, *URDVAH MUKHA SVANASANA / ADHO MUKHA SVANASANA*

Begin in Plank Pose, *Chataranga Dandasana*, a push up position, (Position A). Inhale push the sitting bones back to Down Dog (Position B). Exhale as you drop through Plank Pose to lift the head and chest into Upward Facing Dog and gently look up at the sky or the ceiling (Position C). Remember to drop the shoulders away from the ears. Perform for 10-breaths. Finish with standing for 3-Whisper Breaths.

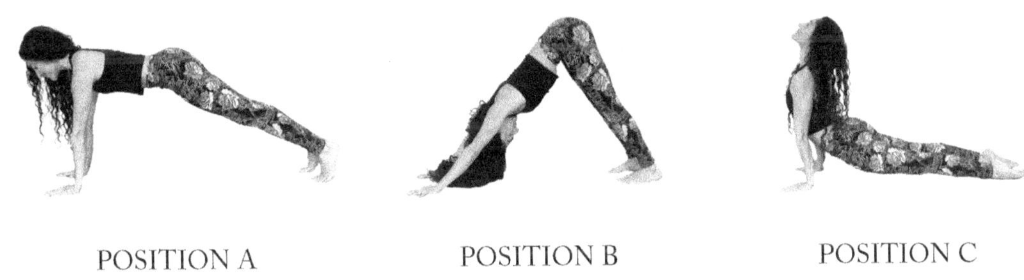

POSITION A   POSITION B   POSITION C

Benefits

This flow energizes and warms the body. Strengthens the arms, shoulders, back and abdominals, and stretches and strengthens both the front and back of the body including the hamstring and ankles and feet. Because of their enormous benefit to the body and ease in movement, these two poses are part of the foundation of most sun salutation series. Performing them on a regular basis will not only benefit your practice immensely, but will put you on the fast track to feeling simultaneously stronger, more flexible, and leaner.

The breath is opposite of normal yogic breathing, which usually is inhaled for chest opening postures.

DETOXIFYING BELLY SQUEEZE

Begin in a comfortable standing position. Take a few deep breaths. Then inhale deeply (Position A), and as you exhale deeply, squeeze the lower belly in as you pump the abdominal muscles, squeezing the stomach in and up as much as you can for as long as you can (Position B). Inhale and relax. Then do a few more breaths with a detoxifying belly squeeze, 2 - 5-breaths total.

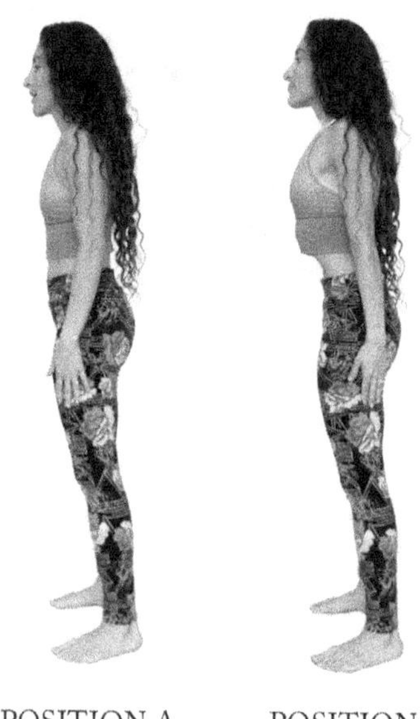

POSITION A   POSITION B

SAVASANA

Relax, release, breath in and out peace for 10 - 20-breaths. You may also use your choice of any of the previously mentioned lessons on Savasana for this session.

HAVE A BLESSED DAY, NAMASTE

Week Six Summary of Poses

5 TIBETAN RITES - 3 WHISPER BREATHS BETWEEN EACH POSE

10 CLOCKWISE SPINS
10 ABDOMINAL LEG LIFTS - TUCK CHIN

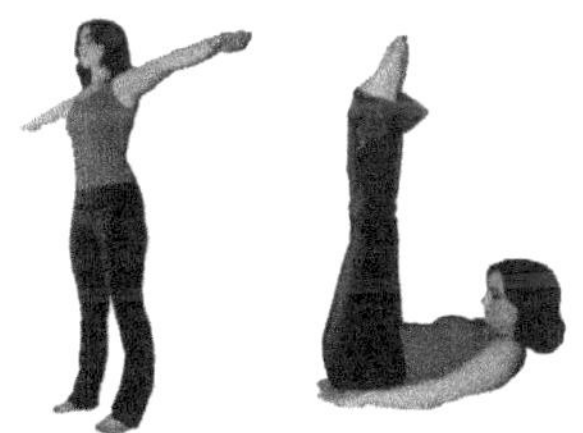

10 CAMEL FLOWS
10 DANDANSA TO BRIDGE

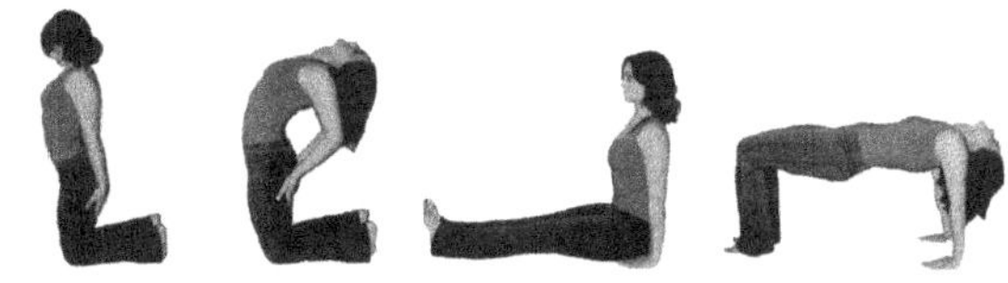

10 UP DOG / DOWN DOG

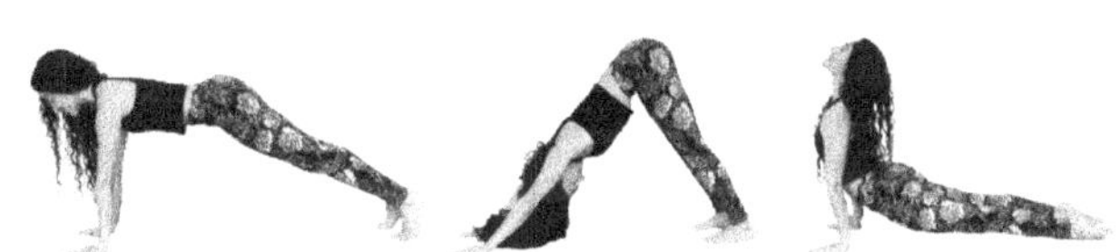

SQUEEZE LOWER BELLY IN - 2 BREATHS

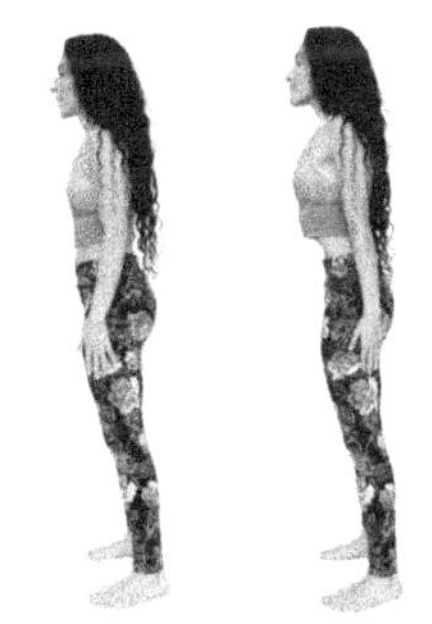

SAVASANA - RELAX, RELEASE, BREATH IN AND OUT PEACE

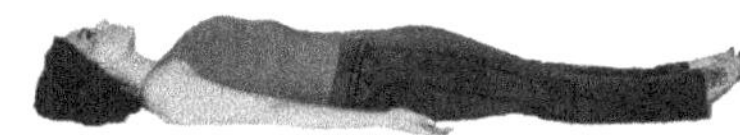

BONUS COMBINED POSES
1.5-HOUR YOGA SESSION

INTRO

The following one-and-half-hour session incorporates all the poses you have learned in this book. After you have mastered ten minutes a day, you could try several ten-minute sessions in one day. For instance, try ten minutes in the morning, then ten minutes before lunch during a lunch break and then ten minutes again in the evening. After you have finished six weeks of ten minutes per day, you should be ready for deeper sessions as time permits. If an hour seems too daunting for you, you could try to combine several weeks' lessons for twenty-minute sessions before you jump to the full hour and a half session. In any case, do not be frightened by the time. When I sit on my mat to begin my practice, ten minutes often turns into thirty. But if I only have time in that moment for ten minutes, it's usually the best ten minutes of my day.

Also, you can use this summary of poses as a guide to develop your own practice. As you develop your personal practice, you'll want to make sure you incorporate twist, forward and back bending postures, abdominal strengthening poses, relaxation poses, sitting poses and Savasana into your sessions. Use this section as a guide to expand your practice, experimenting with various amounts of time during different times of the day that works for you and your body.

DHARMA

How we nourish ourselves daily is essential in expanding our lives or contracting and inhibiting our lives, whichever the case may be. When we starve our bodies of nutrition by eating fake fast foods, full of plastic saturated oils, and animal flesh void of essential nutrients like vitamin C, we become weaker and more constricted. However, Yoga is a nurturing practice and is a key component to expanding how we live in the world when off the mat. When we nourish our lives with invigorating movement, healthy vitamin and mineral infused foods, and happy, compassionate, and successful thoughts, we will truly be living as our empowered, vibrant higher selves.

CROSS LEGGED SITING – 5 Breaths

ABDOMINAL SQUEEZE WITH BREATH OF FIRE – 5 to 10 Breaths

SPINE FLEXES – 10 Breaths each pose

WASHING MACHINE – 10 Breaths

SHOULDER DROPS – 5 Breaths

CROSS LEGGED FORWARD BEND – 5 Breaths each side

CAT / COW POSES – 10 Breaths

MOUNTAIN POSE – 5 Breaths

STRETCH ON TOES – 10 Breaths

SIDE BENDS - 10 Breaths

FORWARD BEND FLOW – 10 Breaths

STANDING FORWARD BEND – 5 Breaths

SHOULDER ROLLS – 5 Breaths forward and back

NECK ROLLS – 3 Breaths rolling right and 3 left

CAT / COW POSES – 10 Breaths

THREAD THE KNEEDLE – 5 Breaths each side

BENT KNEE DOWN DOG – 5 Breaths

COW-CAT-COW-DOWNDOG – 10 Breaths

DOWN DOG – 5 Breaths

PLANK – 5 Breaths

SPINX – 5 Breaths

COBRA FLOW – 5 Breaths

3 SUNSALUTATIONS

SIDE STRETCH – 5 Breaths on each side

WARRIER II POSE – 5 Breaths on each side

TADASANA – 5 Breaths

CHAIR POSE – 5 Breaths

WINDMILL – 10 Breaths

WINDMILL SIDE STRETCH – 6 Breaths

STRADDLE FORWARD BEND – 5 Breaths

MINI SUN SALUTE TO

UPWARD BOW – 5 Breaths

EXTENDED CHILD'S POSE – 5 Breaths

FALLEN LEAF – 5 Breaths

SEATED FORWARD BEND – 5 Breaths

MODIFIED BOAT POSE – 5 Breaths X 3

BOAT POSE – 5 Breaths X 2

STAFF POSE – 5 Breaths

SEATED TWIST – 10 Breaths

ONE LEG SEATED FORWARD BEND JANU SIRASANA – 5 Breaths each side

EASY BRIDGE – 5 Breaths

MODIFIED SHOULDER STAND – 5 Breaths

CRADLE ROCK – 5 Breaths each

RELAXATION POSE – 10-20 Breaths

SATNAM – 5 Breaths

RELEASE INTO POSE – 10 to 20 Breaths

THE BODY

I've included some quick and easy recipes that may also enhance your life and your practice with extra vitamins, minerals, and energy. And just as with the suggestions for finding your own practice that works for you, I encourage you to experiment with these recipes. And to expand your knowledge about yoga and food choices, you may research more yoga books, cookbooks, and other recourses I have listed in the bibliography so that you can make the best choices for you.

If we are what we eat, let us eat healthy, vibrant, energy filled foods, not the dead, plastic-wrapped foods found in grocery stores and fast-food factories. Every day we have choices to make about our wellbeing and the wellbeing of the planet. As we choose life, and healthy, organic foods from local farmers, we not only benefit ourselves with nutrient rich foods but also benefit our local economies. If our dollars have power, it is in how we choose to use this energy daily. Every day is an opportunity to enrich our lives in every way. We do not have to choose options that do not support our wellbeing. If a food does not support our wellbeing, it probably doesn't support a living planet either.

A fellow traveler once told me that he stopped eating fast-food because he'd forgotten a hamburger in his car. And after weeks, it was still, mostly intact. He decided that if bacteria are smart enough not to eat it, humans should be too.

Some of these recipes are my favorites that I create to eat more vibrantly rich greens daily. However, these recipes can be altered to your liking. You can change the fruits in the smoothie to your taste or add other spices to them like cinnamon. I add Garam Masala, an Indian spice blend, to many of my smoothies, especially the melon-based ones. I have also included a soup recipe that can be altered to use with almost any type of soup you are enjoying. If our taste buds and the cells of our bodies are jumping for joy, maybe we will be too. And as we transform the health of our bodies, minds, and spirits, perhaps we are transforming the energy of our planet to benefit all living beings.

"Also, go inside and listen to your body because your body will never lie to you. Your mind will play tricks, but the way you feel in your heart, in your guts, is the truth." – Don Miguel Ruiz

VIBRANT RECIPES

GREEN SMOOTHIE

One of my all-time favorite drinks is a green smoothie. It's not only tremendously healthy; it's amazingly delicious.

Ingredients:

- 3-5 cups of your favorite greens, (spinach, kale, etc.)

- 2 cups Nut, rice, soy, or oat milk

- Fresh or frozen fruit of your choice

- 1 teaspoon vanilla extract

- 1 tablespoon peanut or other nut butter (optional)

- 1 scoop of veggie protein powder

You may use store bought nut, soy, oat, or rice milk. But you can also start with blending a handful of soaked almonds or pine nuts or cashew for a nice nut milk flavor. Soak the nuts for a few hours or overnight. You can use the nut water too. After soaking, blend first then add greens and fruits. I add about a 1/4th blender full of nut milk. Coconut milk is great too.

Next add half a blender full of kale, spinach, sweet potato leaves, or other favorite green. You can even use celery stalks with leaves or carrot tops if you can find them.

I avoid raw collard greens for smoothies because they are spicy and bitter when raw, but you may like this combination of flavors in your smoothies.

Fill the rest of the blender with your favorite fresh or frozen fruits like a banana, blue berries, mangoes, peaches, fresh peeled oranges, etcetera. Mixing different fruits and greens can give you many variations. Any type of berry is usually a good idea. Since berries are considered super foods and are loaded with vital nutrients, any chance to get more of them into our diet is a good one. Adding a banana or mango to your smoothies will ensure that they have a delicious creamy texture.

Add 1 teaspoon vanilla extract (real is better)

You might add some peanut butter or other nut butter for some extra protein, fat and flavor.

And for a more malt like taste, I add a scoop of raw or other veggie protein powder.

Blend until smooth.

Drink immediately. Share with family. Save some for later in a recycled jar. It's best to fill the jars to the top and seal if you want some for the next day.

May your life be sweet, green, and healthy.

Victoria Boutenko's book, *Green for Life*, propelled my own journey into the world of green smoothies. Her book lists savory recipes and all sorts of variations on green smoothies. But the most important part is that it presents a thorough scientific argument for the importance of greens in our daily diet.

EASY NUTTY OAT MILK

This is a quick way to make homemade vegan milk for smoothies, coffee, tea, puddings etc.

Ingredients:

- 2 cups nuts

- 5 or more cups water

- 1 cup oatmeal

- 1/2 teaspoon vanilla (optional)

- 1 banana (optional)

- 1/8 teaspoon turmeric powder (optional)

- Pinch black pepper (optional)

- Nut bag for straining

Soak raw almonds and or any other nuts you like, for instance, pecans, walnuts, cashews for a few hours. I usually drain this water because the nuts will release digestive blocking enzymes in the water and become more nutritionally viable after soaking. Then add a cup or so of oatmeal, optional drop or so of vanilla and if you like a banana. You may add an optional sprinkle of turmeric, and a pinch of black pepper because black pepper is important for metabolizing the amazing benefits of turmeric. This makes this a yogi Golden Milk. Next, fill the blender with water up to the top of the mixture; you may add more above.

After blending until smooth, use a nut bag to strain the milk into a bowl and then pour into a bottle for use. It's creamy and delicious. And if you omit the vanilla and banana, you can use this milk for creamy savory sauces and to make vegan cheeses. I often save the nut pulp to add to muffins or vegan cheese.

SOUPY SALAD

Ingredients:

- ½ cup shredded lettuce or spinach of your choice

- 1/4 cup shredded cabbage

- ¼ cup shredded carrots, beets, zucchini, squash, and or other veggies

- 1-2 tablespoons sliced or diced red or green onion

- ¼ cup diced tomato

- 1-2 cups veggie broth

- 1 teaspoon Braggs Liquid Aminos

- 1-2 tablespoons coconut milk (optional)

- Indian, Thai, or spice blend of your choice

This is also one of my all-time favorite discoveries. I begin with warm homemade veggie stock and add my favorite spices. The flavor I choose depends on the mood I'm in, which usually leans toward Thai, green curry coconut. Another staple is lemon, cayenne pepper and some Braggs, a liquid beefy soy based amino blend found in most grocery stores. You can use store bought veggie stock if you don't have any handy. However, I have included an easy recipe to make your own veggie stock.

Prepare a bowl of shredded lettuce, grated carrots, grated zucchini, green onion, sprouts, diced tomato, maybe some sliced yellow squash. You can add any raw veggies or salad fixings that you'd like to your bowl. Now pour the warm broth over the bowl of salad and enjoy the warmth of soup with the healthy delicious enzymes from the raw veggies. Yum!

I try to come up with as many ways as possible to eat more raw food. Organic raw food is rich in the vitamins, minerals, and enzymes our bodies need. Even though some cooked vegetables are considered more easily digestible, like kale and broccoli, in general, cooked food is inferior to raw fruits and vegetables and usually contains no enzymes necessary for digestion. So, including plenty of raw foods in our diets is essential for a healthy, happy, holy mind, body and soul.

I encourage you to experiment with these recipes to find what works for you. And to alternate greens at least every few days in your green smoothies. These two enlightening books, *Rainbow Green Live-Food Cuisine* by Gabriel Cousins, M.D., and the Sun Food Diet Success System by David Wolf provide more thorough explainations of the benefits of eating raw foods.

PLAN A DAY RETREAT AT HOME

If you feel like you have too much work, not enough work, never enough money and neither the time or funds for a yoga retreat in Costa Rico, then a day retreat, or even a weekend retreat at home or at an economical ashram or retreat center, or an inexpensive day in nature may be just the thing. There are countless websites that advertise the best retreat centers. Almost any yoga or meditation retreat center would likely be amazingly refreshing, but doing research and reading reviews and even asking your local yoga teacher for a recommendation is a way to find the best one for you.

However, taking a weekend home retreat right where you are, may be just what your mind, body, and soul need. For a home retreat, if possible, turn cellphones off the night before to prevent unwanted distractions. Many may have loved ones who require more available communication, like children, elderly parents, or friends with special needs. However, if these practitioners can turn their phones off even for a few hours during the day to concentrate on their yoga practice, or take an undisturbed hot bath, the benefits may be profound. It can be stressful to try to relax, knowing that at any moment a device may be sounding.

Also, if your home needs some de-cluttering, you do not necessarily need to declutter like Marie Kondo suggests in her famous book, *The Life Changing Magic of Tidying Up*, to feel a sense of stress-free freedom; you may simply need to remove distracting items from eyesight. If you see unfinished tasks, like sorting mail for instance, this may cause stress and take valuable mental and physical energy away from your day retreat. I have a box that I keep mail that does not need immediate attention, but I might want to revisit. Your home or your life does not need to be perfect to take a day, weekend, or a few hours for yourself.

Plan to drink lots of extra water to help detoxify the body while you are healing. Many cleanses like the one in the famous *Master Cleanser* by Stanley Burroughs suggest drinking distilled water to expedite the cleansing process. But slices of lemon or orange in filtered or spring water may work just as well. It is important to drink more water during this time. And in general, after a yoga session, a massage, or any form of physical detoxification, it's a good idea to drink a glass of water immediately after the session and extra water to help detoxify the body and remove any toxins that this session has assisted the body in dislodging and releasing.

Also be mindful of the sights and sounds in your environment. For instance, to add a bit of decor to the giant black beckoning screen, I sometimes cover my television screen with a beautiful cloth or scarf. Rather than listening to popular music on the raideo, I also listen to soothing yoga music during yoga sessions and during relaxing days. Music has the ability influence feelings of sadness, depression, and stress, or it can help to heal what ails us and lift our spirits. Once in Graduate school, I was in a car listening to a popular CD with my roommate, who suffered from depression. This was her favorite CD. After a few songs, I was on the verge of tears. I realized that this music may be competent and skilled, but it was severely depressing. I told her that this was not helping her depression and that she should consider listening to more uplifting music.

The main idea is that a day retreat at home should be simple, uncluttered, relaxing, refreshing, healing, and rejuvenating. It's not about overdoing; it's about opening our lives to the sound of our breath, to the unencumbered stretching of the body, and to the simple taste of lemon water and fresh strawberries.

IDEAS FOR BEGINNING AND ENDING YOUR REFRESHING DAY

Morning

Upon awakening, drink a cup of warm lemon water or herbal tea. I like to sit outside if the weather permits and sip this slowing while gazing at the sky. When you finish your cup, you may walk barefoot in the grass, a technique called grounding. There are many who do this to reconnect to the Earth's healing electromagnetic energy. By gently placing the feet, taking one step per breath, you can make this ritual a regular morning meditation.

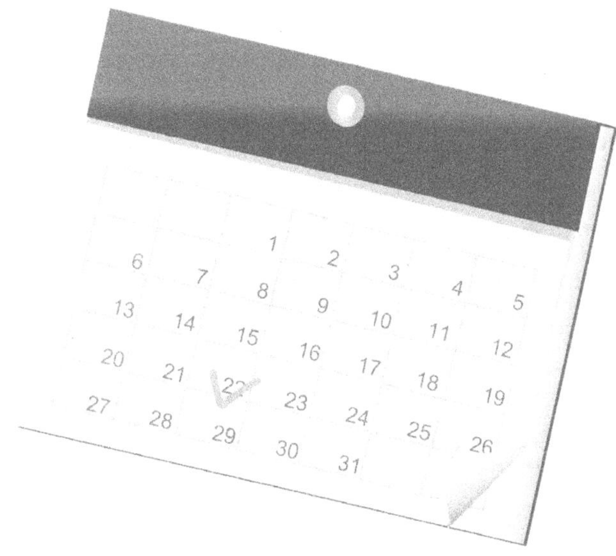

After tea and grounding, you may indulge in a cool rejuvenating shower. Yogi Bhajan recommends taking cold showers to invigorate the nervous system. I must admit; this is difficult to do but feels amazing. The cold water opens blood vessels near the skin and turns on the body's natural heating system. A cool or cold shower is invigorating. There are also gyms and spas that offer cold dips in addition to the traditional steam rooms, saunas, and jacuzzis. The health benefits of cold water are nearly unlimited. About ten minutes or less is usually sufficient to jump start this pleasantly shocking, heating, healing process.

Another water cleanse is a neti. And If you are feeling a little under-the-weather because of allergies or change of season, it's even better to rinse these seasonal toxins from nasal passages. Boil water first, then fill the neti pot with warm water and a pinch of sea salt to rinse the nose and sinuses. Wait until the water is body temperature before rinsing. Tilt the head and pour the fluid into one nostril. Breath through the mouth or not at all for a moment. Let the water run out of the other nostril. Do a little in each side, maybe a few times. I usually inhale a little into the sinus cavity to rinse this area and blow my nose really well after rinsing. There are also salt-water nasal cleanses available in drug stores.

After cleansing, especially If you live in a dry area, you may lubricate the inside of the nose with drops of sesame oil by carefully applying the oil with the pinky fingers. This is also helpful in winter months when heaters can dry the nasal passages, which can prevent the cilia, the hairs in the nose, from properly doing their job of collecting microbes before these uninvited particles and organisms enter the body, where they can wreak havoc.

After cleansing, you might prepare a small bottle of warm coconut or almond oil with a few drops of lavender oil for a relaxing face, neck, and / or foot massage. There are many books on massage, but in general, for the face, massage center outward, focusing on the brow area, temples, under the cheek bones, and anywhere you feel tension. Massaging up and down the neck and then gently pressing any tight muscles can be very effective. And for the feet, you might also use a roller or ball or simply a gulf ball can be wonderful to workout tension on soles of the feet. Perhaps nurturing the soles of our feet is a powerful practice in honoring our souls.

After this wake-up gentle detox massage, it's time to drink a large glass of lemon water. The lemon not only adds wonderful flavor to water but adds vitamin C and is good for digestion. Stanley Burroughs' book, *The Master Cleanser*, explains more of the details of lemon water. When cleansing the body, and after yoga and a massage, drinking extra water is even more important as the body is flushing out the toxins that may have been released during the massage.

It's time for some gentle yoga to begin your day. Choose week one or another week's lesson from this book. If you combine poses on your own, make sure you include side bend, forward bend, and a variation of back bend poses. If you are feeling tension in the shoulders, you could include shoulder shrugs for instance. And breathing deeply into twists is a way to detox and massage internal organs.

After yoga, sitting on a zafu or a comfortable cushion is a great way to feel supported for
a 10-30 minute meditation. Meditations can be practiced lying down or in a comfortable
chair; however, try not to fall asleep. You could practice any of the meditations in this book
or one of your choosing. If you are Catholic, you may find healing and peace by reciting
the rosary prayers. You may recite a Hindu prayer, such as the Gayatri Mantra for healing.
One of my favorite mantras is the Nicheren Buddhist chant for world peace, Nam Myoho
Renge Kyo. These mantras can be audible or simply recited in the mind with the breath.

Chanting helps to release the thoughts that can plague our peace of mind so that we can
have a moment of reprieve from our relentless ego, which is in constant motion, within our
fear-based mind.

Nicheren Buddhist practitioners think of chanting like
brushing their teeth. Chanting helps to rid the mind of
the debris of outdated ideas that can cause tarter on
our brains and even create pain like cavities that are
constantly triggered by the events of daily life.

"To free yourself of the invisible ties of karma, to achieve
"karmic escape velocity," you must increase the power
of your life force until it becomes greater than the force of
karmic pull." - Tina Turner in *Happiness Becomes You*.

Especially in the spring and summer, I love to start my day with a light energizing meal,
like fresh fruits and nuts or, a favorite, sliced fresh fruit over shredded lettuce sprinkled with
fresh lemon juice, served with a side of warm ginger tea. If this is not how you'd start your
day normally, all the better. If you plan a special day at home for yourself, changing your
normal routine will help you to realize the peace and healing you are choosing to create.

And if you want to add meditation to your meal, close the eyes and focus on the taste
and smell of each sip of tea and small bite of fruit. I notice when I am rushing through

my day, I often eat without intention, simply chewing some fuel, so I can keep going. But the delight of allowing our taste buds an opportunity to celebrate is amazing.

Reading a spiritual and uplifting book or article can be next on the agenda. There is a bibliography of suggested readings at the end of this book to help you begin the journey of *Svadhyaya*, self-study. As we read spiritual, positive, and truthful texts, we become more aware in our daily lives. This also might be the encouragement we need to continue our cleanse or to break free from "stuckage" as I call it, the muscle or life spasms that keep us stuck in old patterns. Self-study can also inspire us to take stock of our life and choices, and in yoga terms, to do this without judgment.

There are three main principles in SGI Nichiren Daishonin's Buddhism, faith, practice, and study. Studying Buddhist texts is essential to maintain the momentum of practice, which in turn creates proof in practitioners' daily lives and therefore enhances their faith in the practice. Faith, practice, and study work as a trinity together.

Afternoon

During my daily life, but especially for a raw food cleanse, I like to have healthy snacks like carrots, apples, tangerines, grapes, nuts, peanut butter, and celery sticks handy. Snacks that are easily digestible and low in calories are usually best. You can check on the internet for more foods that are low in calories, like sliced cucumber, etc.

Avoiding driving a car is ideal, but if you must drive to a park or someplace else, be present. I sometimes practice this by thinking, "Hands on wheel. Foot on break. Gliding in neutral," etc., calming thoughts that take my attention back ot the present moment. I often smile when I practice this because it feels a little silly. Many cities have beautiful parks, but if you are fortunate enough to have nature nearby, great, but an observant walk in your neighborhood can be just as good. I like to walk a little slower on these days, really observing the birds, the trees, and the sky. Again, if you must drive, relax, be at peace, and try not to drive too fast or too far.

A delicious, fruity, green smoothie is great for a cleans or just to have handy any time. Enjoying a giant green smoothie for lunch with your favorite fruits and greens - kale or spinach or both is refreshing and invigorating. See the suggested recipe in this book or find one in "Green for Life," or on line. You can use your imagination, by adding cinnamon, garum masala, pumpkin pie spices or other spices. One of my favorites includes mango juice with coconut vanilla kefir.

I like to sit outside on my veranda and read a spiritual or uplifting Buddhist book on these refreshing days. But you might enjoy Christian, Hindu, Islamic or other religious stories or simply an uplifting article or book. Even a good fiction book can be refreshing as long as it's not violent. There is a list of suggested reading in "My Favorites" at the end of this book for ideas on learning more about yoga, meditation, mindfulness, and Buddhism. Any of these books would enhance a refreshing retreat. Keeping the mind calm and free of societies' disorder and often false negativity is important to cleanse the mind and soul of unwanted debris and falsehoods. Any ideas of lack or negative ideas about your or anyone else's potential should be avoided. If your mind is cluttered with such ideas, that is more reason to fill it with some essential vital nutrients of a good uplifting book or story. What we consume in our bodies and minds is often what we will experience in our lives.

And if you are so inclined, playing a guitar or a small drum or even a tiny child-sized keyboard can be relaxing and fun. If you do this without judgment, you might be amazed at the sounds you can create. I know I am when I practice this. However, if you are not like me, and do not have an assortment of musical instruments, then listing to yoga or relaxing music is a way to refresh the ears, mind, and soul with pleasing sounds.

While you are listening to soothing music, if you feel like moving, dancing is yet another way to heal and feel rejuvenated. Again, you don't have to worry about how you are moving; stretching, and hopping, whatever feels good to you is the way to create joy and happiness in every cell of your body. Whatever afternoon activity you choose, make a gentle effort to be in the moment, practicing non-judgment, free for a moment to just be. Dancing is also a great way to release stuck-age and energize your body, mind, and soul. Perhaps this is why indigenous people from around the world use dancing as part of their healing and spiritual practices.

Choose a more advanced week's lesson for some invigorating afternoon yoga, for instance week five or six. Again, if you combine poses on your own, make sure you do the appropriate counter poses. There is a lesson on combining postures in this book.

You might want to take a nap after another long meditation 10-30 minutes or more. You could repeat your morning meditation and mantra or simply sit quietly becoming aware of the breath, breathing in the moment.

It's easy to feel like just breathing is a waste of time, especially if you are like me. I'm usually juggling many thoughts and activities, from grading classes, attending Buddhist events, going to yoga classes, to meeting friends at publishing events, etc. There is also money, cars, children, and jobs to keep our minds on full throttle. But taking these few moments for ourselves on these precious days can be the beginning to a more regular daily practice of mindfulness.

In addition, the benefits to, not only our health and emotional wellbeing of this clearing the mind practice, but to our mental health, are enormous. With so many people suffering from dementia, depression, attention deficit disorder etc., there may have never been a better time to keep the mind fresh and clean, so that it does not short circuit. There is a lot of research in the field of mindfulness happening in psychology and neurology that is showing promising results in regards to the benefits of meditation.

In Presences, How Mindfulness and Meditation Shape Our Brain, Mind, and Life, Paul Verhaeghen, likens meditation to a mental gym. Keeping our minds strong, flexible and sharp may help us navigate the world in more joyful, positive ways. Buddhists liken negative functions, like depression, or negative events to a form of poison, and when we overcome these obstacles joyfully, helping humanity to blossom in a new or seemingly extraordinary way, we are turning poison into medicine. I recently saw a one-woman-play, *The Mask of Joy,* written and performed by Julie Turner, where a disabled woman, who had once been a prima-ballerina had fallen from the roof of her apartment, down six floors into an elevator shaft, where a janitor found her. She woke up days later in the hospital, listening to doctors say that she would never walk again. She used the power of her mind to overcome this seemingly impossible obstacle.

However, Verhaeghen also warns that even though mindfulness is showing positive results for patients with sleep disorders, anxiety, and other illnesses, and in the field of pain management, it may not be a "Buddha pill." I think expecting magic is not the answer, in yoga, in meditation, in a Buddhist practice or in life. However, taking action, and using our minds as tools for healing, not only ourselves, but our communities, and ultimately this planet, is the answer.

Think of this day as a day of discovery, a day to discover more about you, the you that you did not know existed, or the you that you haven't seen in a long time. This is an opportunity for self-discovery. It's an opportunity to be creative, or simply to be at one with the breath, this moment, the Earth. On these days especially, I like to keep a journal to write about my day. I used to have more time for self-reflection, but now my days are full of helping others self-reflect, which is yet another reason why a day or weekend retreat is even more important. I often have revelations or new creative ideas after a long meditation or chanting session. I see this as divine inspiration.

And if you have begun your cleanse avoiding caffeine, be prepared for a mild or severe headache, depending on your addiction level to caffeine. If this happens, try peppermint essential oil rubbed on the temples, and while you are meditating, breath in the peppermint, which will help heal those aching receptors of the brain. If this fails, and your headache becomes worse, go ahead and have a cup of Joe. This should alleviate the pain.

Evening

A spinach salad with sesame, lemon, olive oil or other salad dressing with an assortment of veggies like bell peppers, celery, green onion, tomato, and maybe some added raisins, or pear or strawberry slices is a good way to end the day. Serve dinner with your favorite hot tea or fresh vegetable or fruit juice. As usual, during a yoga cleanse, practice being present even in the eating and drinking process, really focusing on the pleasant sensations on the tongue. This is what makes a strawberry taste divine.

Continue reading that spiritual book you started this morning, or select a new one from the list in the back of the book. You might also take out your journal and write about your vision of happiness. Writing has a power all on its own. It's a physical manifestation of our dreams and desires. As the pen sets ink on a page or fingers move on a keyboard, we are dropping our dreams on screen of paper. And once we have written something down, it increases its potency and our connection to Universal Consciousness or God, thereby increasing the likelihood of its manifestation in the physical world.

Gentle yoga stretches before going to bed is a great way to end any day, but especially a stay home yoga retreat day. Breathing deeply and holding postures for a little extended time in, for instance, *Janu Sirsansana* and a counter pose, *Matsyasana*, is a great way to help you fall asleep and get a good night's rest. You could take a minute or more breathing into poses. Remember to choose counter poses with both sides of the body and light postures, nothing to strenuous or energizing.

For the final meditation of the day, imagine the day you had today and how it flowed beautifully. Feel and see your accomplishments. Now visualize your next day in the world with the same sense of wonder, love and possibility. Whatever your job is, imagine yourself at work feeling refreshed, invigorated, and excited about helping others and facing any obstacles with compassion and determination.

Before bed, drinking a cup of lemon or chamomile tea will help you unwind for a rejuvenating night's sleep so that you can have the best night of your life in blissful relaxation.

Taking a retreat doesn't have to be expensive or a big ordeal, and how wonderful it is to take this precious time for yourself. If you are tired and worn-down from life, then you will not be able to be of service to those you love, and ultimately to humanity. Therefore, finding a few moments in your day to rejuvenate yourself can create unexpected wonders in your life. When we are taking care of ourselves, other people feel this rising energy. With clear minds, healthy bodies, and empowered souls, we can make wise decisions for ourselves and others.

So many, often-dangerous, mistakes are made by people who are tired. People want and need to do their best. A truck driver needs to be well rested to drive hundreds of miles a day; a lawyer needs to be invigorated to help clients make the best decisions or inspired to recite the most moving closing arguments. Doctors need to be sharp to help save lives. Teachers need to be excited about presenting new ideas and fresh perspectives to their students. The list goes on. No matter what your profession, being your absolute best is crucial. And taking precious time for yourself is one way to ensure that you are functioning at your best.

FIVE-MINUTE BREAKS

Wherever you are, at an office, in a warehouse, in a shop, a five-minute break can help focus and invigorate the next few hours. You can use a timer on your phone so that you are not distracted with thoughts of time and can completely enjoy your five minutes.

One Options

❀ Find a quiet place if one is available; if not, find a mostly secluded area.

❀ Sit or lie down if that is available; if not, you can stand.

❀ Close your eyes and focus on your breath.

❀ Begin to inhale and exhale as deeply as possible.

❀ Imagine inhaling to the fingers and toes. As you exhale imagine any tension leaving your body with the breath.

❀ Finally enjoy a sip of your favorite beverage, a cup of calming herbal tea, or a water with lemon, or even a cup of coffee.

Sometimes in the afternoon when there is a lull in energy, my tendency is to reach for caffeine as a pick me up, and that's fine, but instead, when I focus on breathing or movement of some kind, I usually feel much better.

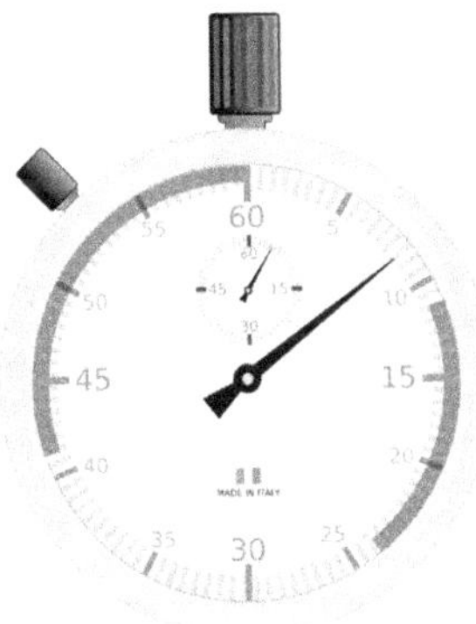

Another Option

❀ At your desk practice some spine flexes and gentle twist.

❀ Take a brisk walk around the office or walk around the block.

❀ Stand and do a few of Windmill Pose.

❀ Stretch up onto the toes and stretch the hands over head.

❀ Do any yoga poses that suit your style and work environment.

Option Three

❀ Find a quiet and mostly secluded area where you can unroll your yoga mat.

❀ Practice some Cat / Cow and Downward Facing Dogs.

❀ Then move to a few standing poses like Proud Warrior and Side bends.

❀ Chose whatever poses or routines that suit you.

The idea that rejuvenation or relaxation requires hours of our time is absolutely false. Hours is great, but in our fast-paced world, not many people have hours to stretch and breathe throughout the day. So, taking a few minutes to thank your body for all that it does and to center your mind can be like diving into a blue lagoon of peace anytime you like. And even if your dip is short, it's still cool and refreshing.

SUGGESTIONS FOR TRAVELING

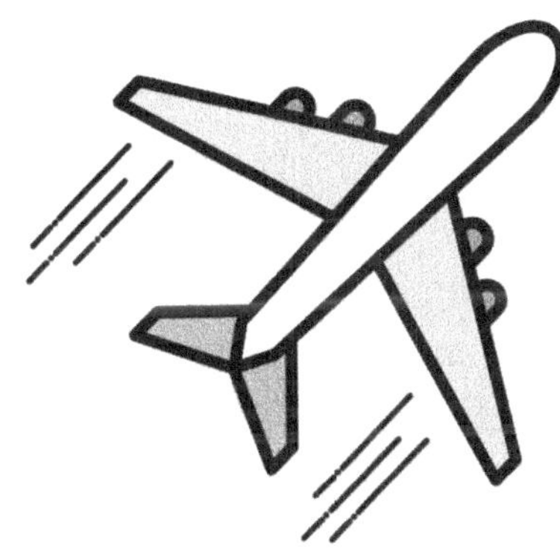

Traveling can be a fun adventure, but sitting on a plane or in a car for hours can cause our bodies to be stiff and sore. Fortunately, there are simple ways to alleviate a lot of that soreness.

❀ Practice spine Flexes in your seat

❀ Relax your upper body into a forward fold over your bent legs

❀ When you do get to stand up, reach the arms above the head and stretching the entire body long.

❀ If you are in an airport or at a rest stop on the road, practice some Windmills and Forward Bend Flows

❀ When you arrive at your hotel or destination, practice your favorite ten-minute session before heading out for the day or evening.

Don't forget to pack a travel yoga mat or sticky travel yoga towel so that you can continue to practice your ten-minutes every day. This way you will have more energy for the activities you love and more enthusiasm in doing them.

HOW TO CREATE YOUR OWN SESSION AND PRACTICE

There will be days when you feel like Cat / Cow is all you need. You have forward and back bending all in one. Adding a few strenthening and stretching Down Dogs can energize your day. But truly, you can choose three minutes, five minutes, fifteen minutes, or two hours' to practice postures, meditation, and chanting. It's up to you.

If you include a few back bending, forward bending, breathing, and meditation postures, you will feel more centered and balanced than before you began. And you will have more energy and enthusiasm for each precious moment of your life.

Local yoga classes are also a great way to continue to develop your practice and to learn new postures and challenge yourself to do more than you thought you could ever do. I continue to attend yoga classes, usually because I enjoy the sound of another person's soothing voice gently guiding me into realizing my best self. And I continue to develop my practice in the process.

Find instructors who guide you and are not afraid to gently adjust your body to achieve the correct posture.

MORE TIPS FOR A LONG YOGA LIFE

GARLIC

The many wonders of garlic cannot be overstated. The Healing Power of Garlic by Paul Bergner lists some of the gems of garlic as cancer prevention, lowering blood pressure, boosting the immune system, and resisting colds and flu symptoms.

My grandfather, who suffered from arteriosclerosis, used to eat daily doses of the flower called the "stinky rose." He, not only, did not have to worry about vampires, but he never had a heart attack.

From research and my own observations, cooking garlic eliminates some of its healing potency. When I'm feeling a little puffy in my face from allergies or a sudden change in the weather, raw garlic is usually included in my healing regime. To start my day, I may chop a few cloves into tiny pieces and spread them with vegan butter or sliced avocado on a slice of sprouted whole grain bread. Later, I will chop a clove or two and add this to a bowl of soup or whatever I am eating.

Recently, while a friend, who refused to eat the stinky flowers, took weeks to fully recover from flu symptoms, I was completely healed in only two days. Once, I felt warm and energized and healed in only two hours after I mixed two cloves with homemade spring rolls. Not only was this delicious, but it worked.

Garlic is natures natural antibiotic. It's cheap and abundant and has none of the negative side effects of pharmaceutical antibiotics. Most scholars agree that garlic has been used as a medicine for over 7,000 years, and according to the National Institute of Health and the Egyptian text, Codex Ebers, garlic was widely prescribed by doctors for a variety of maladies in ancient Egypt. And if you are concerned about having the dreaded garlic breath (nothing compared to the flu) simply eat a few sprigs of parsley or mint. However, if I am feeling under the weather, I think it's a good idea that people stay a little distance away from me, so I'm not afraid of a little garlic dragon breath.

Humans, like most primates, do not have the ability to make or synthesize their own vitamin C in their bodies. We must eat lots of vitamin C in our diet since we cannot create it. The benefits of vitamin C rich foods are vast. The National Health Society in the United Kingdom sums vitamin C up as follows; "helping to protect cells and keeping them healthy, maintaining healthy skin, blood vessels, bones, and cartilage, and helping with wound healing. The National Institute of Health in the United States list pages of benefits for vitamin C. Let us suffice to say that we cannot live healthy, happy, holy lives without consuming vitamin C rich foods.

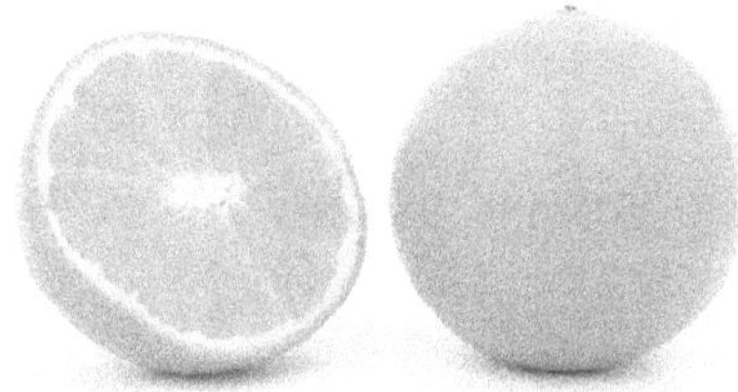

There are vast resources on the Internet and books dedicated to this one subject. I encourage you to research. Ultimately, every meal should include vitamin C rich foods, like any of the orange variety, lemons, green leafy vegetables, tomato, carrots, broccoli, avocado and an abundance of other fruits and vegetables.

Vitamin C rich foods are beautifully abundant, orange, lemon, Brussel sprouts, kale, tomatoes, bell pepper, grapefruit, potatoes, cauliflower, cantaloupe, papaya, strawberries, broccoli, mango, cabbage, guava, and so much more.

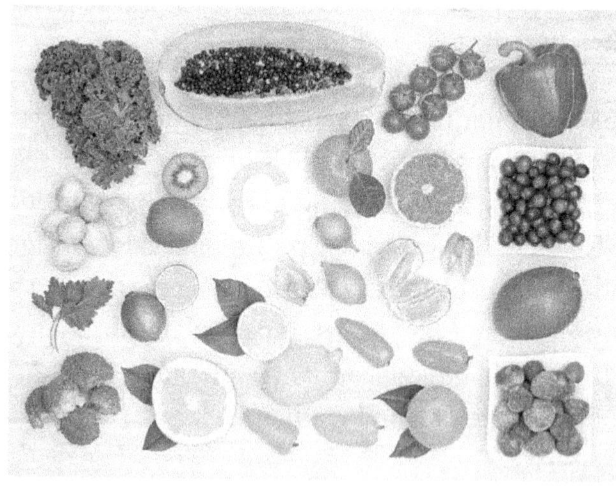

CHLORAPHYLL

Chlorophyll is found in green leaves and distilled in bottles in health food stores to be dropped on the tongue or added to water or a smoothie. It is commonly touted to lower our risk of cancer exponentially. According to the Global Healing Center, chlorophyll helps control cravings, reduces body order, encourages healing, promotes the cleansing of carcinogens from the body, protects DNA against fried foods, is a super potent antioxidant, has been promising in cancer therapy, is effective against Candida infections, relieves redness and swelling and promotes healthy iron levels. So, eat all the greens your heart desires.

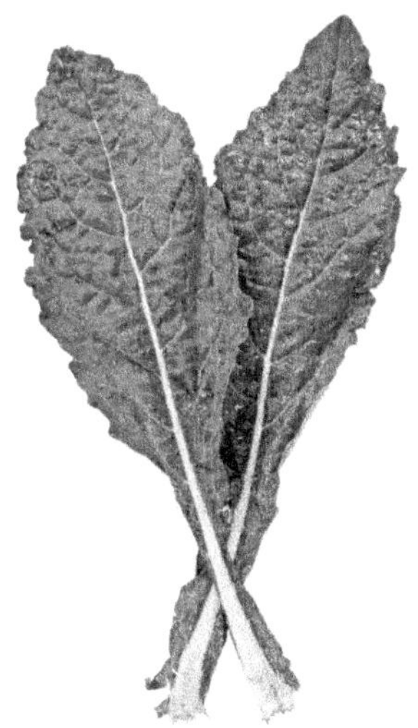

I eat a big leafy salad with almost every meal. If I eat an organic, cruelty free, from my local farmers market, fried in coconut oil egg, I serve this on top of a giant balsamic or lemon and olive oil green salad. It's delicious. If I make a vegan scrambled tofu egg sautéed with lots of veggies, I serve this dish over a bed of greens as well. I encourage you to try to find as many ways as possible to eat more of a variety and more of an abundance of greens.

The book "Green for Life" by Victoria Boutenko is a great
summery of why humans should eat more greens.

FRESH JUICE

Jack Le Layne made juicing a household word, but he had his own struggles to overcome, which lead him to be the fitness guru that he became. At fifteen, after meeting Paul Bragg at a seminar, he went home and prayed, "Please give me the willpower and intestinal fortitude to refrain from eating wrong, lifeless, dead foods when the urge comes over me. God, please give me the strength to exercise when I don't feel like it." Jack LaLanne lived a healthy, energizing life and was an example of how vibrant people can be throughout their sixties, seventies and even eighties if they eat life enriching foods and move the body through proper exercise.

One of his ways for infusing an abundance of energy and nutrition into the body quickly was to drink lots of fresh squeezed juices. There are many others who have documented great successes with juicing. Dr. Max Gerson in the 1920s in his groundbreaking book, A Cancer Therapy, told how he cured all fifty of his patients with a juicing, herbal tea, and raw food regiment. His daughter, Charlotte Gerson was a living example of the healing center, the Gerson Institute, that she founded in her father's name. Please see the bibliography for information on her books and on her father's ground-breaking book that describes his experiment and success.

An easy juice recipe is the Trinity. It's simply apples, carrots, and celery. If you purchase a juicer, usually a recipe pamphlet will be included with the product. A slow juicer is a better because it does less heating of the fruits and veggies in the process, but any fresh juicer is better than none. And if you are afraid that you will waste money on the juicer, then try buying fresh squeezed juice from your local health food store before you make that commitment.

In our fast-paced world, taking the time to clean and prepare fruits and vegetables for juicing and then clean the juicer itself can be a daunting task. For this reason, I go through phases where I buy juice at the store, sometimes even a good, processed brand if fresh is not readily available, and then there are times when I have my Champion out on the counter and my citrus juicer ready to go.

Finding more ways to squeeze in more time for yourself and enjoy more healthy foods does not have to be difficult. If we put our mind, body, and souls first, the rest will follow.

RAW FOOD

As I have mentioned earlier, raw food is living food with all its nutritional properties intact, complete with living digestive enzymes. Cooked food is mostly void of essential enzymes for digestion and in most cases is lower in nutritional quality than food in its raw, natural state. To digest cooked foods, our bodies must create enzymes from its own resources rather than relying on the natural enzymes in raw food. Humans are the only species on the earth that cook their food.

There are many books on raw food, but a famous one is *Rainbow Green Live-Food Cuisine* by Gabriel Cousins, M.D. In this book, Doctor Cousin's not only explains the dangers of cooked, genetically engineered, and irradiated foods, but also includes charts on vitamins in foods, benefits of natural farming, photos of healthy cells after raw vegan meal and acidic blood cells after consuming an acid inducing meal like those made with animal products. One of the best features are the many recipes on raw vegan meals created by the Tree of Life Café chefs.

Reducing the amount of cooked foods you eat and replacing this with raw food will greatly enhance your wellbeing in an abundance of ways. You will not only have better digestion, reduce your risk of all known diseases, but will be happier and healthier. And who knows maybe by living a healthier and happier life, more in line with compassion, nature, and how humans were created to be, we might also be a little holier. Here's to being the happiest, healthiest, holiest humans we can be.

CASHEWS

Cashews are a great natural remedy for depression. Evidently, a handful of cashews per day are equivalent to the effects of a daily dosage of Prozac. Go nuts on nuts! They're a healthy source of fat and protein. And you can eat them raw in their unadulterated version for optimum benefits.

SEA SALT BODY SCRUB

Sea salt is naturally detoxifying for the skin. I make my own scrubs by using sea salt from the grocery store and combining this in a jar with a few drops of my favorite essential oil, usually lavender because it such a versatile oil. Drop the oil in the salt and shake the jar to mix well. Now, you're ready for a healing shower. Just before I've finished my shower, I step out of the water to apply the salt scrub. I perform a little Pranic Healing meditation while my body is covered in salt that is great for clearing energy. I imagine all the toxic energy of anger, fear, exposure to toxins from substances or people, or resistance to moving forward is a dark blob leaving my aura and flowing down the drain. Remember to rinse the salt off well before getting out of the shower. To make your skin glow even more and feel smooth and soft, follow the salt scrub by applying sesame and coconut oil to the skin.

NATURAL BODY AND FACE OIL

If you can't eat a product, you shouldn't put it on your skin. Many major cosmetic brands contain numerous carcinogens, known to cause cancer. Rather than change these harmful formulas, some of these companies have opted to create foundations that benefit pink ribbon runs in order to counterbalance the harmful effects of causing cancer to millions of unsuspecting women.

Fortunately, making your own products at home is easy and much less expensive than buying chemical laden products that cause cancer. For my body oil, I use food grade coconut oil, sesame oil, almond oil, and a little grape seed oil. Then I add a little vitamin E, vitamin A, and a few drops of lavender oil to this mixture. I sometimes add shay butter or natural shea butter lotion as well. You can use other essential oils that are beneficial for your skin like orange or bergamot. I usually use the same mixture for my face. I might add a natural sunscreen product on top of my face and body if I'm going to be in the sun. However, coconut oil is also a mild sunscreen. I often receive random, unsolicited complements on my skin, so I know I'm doing something right.

There are many things in life that we cannot control, but what we choose to put on our bodies and in our bodies is thankfully not one of them.

A basic recipe for face and body oil is below. You can also find many recipes online on natural, do-it-yourself make up recipes and natural cosmetic brands. I learned about strawberries as a natural rouge when I was a child model for a department store. It really works. I have used fresh squeezed blackberry juice mixed with some alkaline green powder to make amazing mascara. Even if you just experiment for fun to see what works, you are learning and communicating to your skin and body that you care. These projects can also be fun for the whole family. My nieces have marveled at the mixological creations we've made together.

To make half a blender of natural body and face oil:

1. Fill 1/4th of the blender with coconut oil.

2. Fill the next 1/8th of the blender with sesame and almond oil.

3. Fill the next 1/8th of the blender with slivers of shea butter and coconut butter (optional emollient).

4. Add about 2 tablespoons each of jojoba, vitamin E oil, and vitamin A oil.

5. Add about 20 drops of lavender essential oil.

6. (Optional) add drops of other healthy oils like argon, vitamin C oil, and hyaluronic acid, bergamot essential oil and orange or neroli essential oil.

7. Blend until the ingredients are thoroughly mixed and creamy. Test the texture before bottling, especially if you used shea or coconut butter.

8. Pour into small jars, add the lids, and, to preserve the ingredients, store in the back of the refrigerator until you are ready to use.

So that the ingredients are not too cold or hard, usually the day before use, I take a jar out of the refrigerator. I use small mason jars or clean and reuse other used small glass jars. It's important that you can reach the bottom of the jar to get every last moisturizing, wonderful, magical drop out.

Find a community that resonates with you. Human beings are social creatures and need the exchange of positive energy that community provides. One way is to find people in your chosen field who can lift you to new levels. Choose friends who support your dreams with encouragement and have dreams of their own. Usually, people who have dreams want to help others who have dreams.

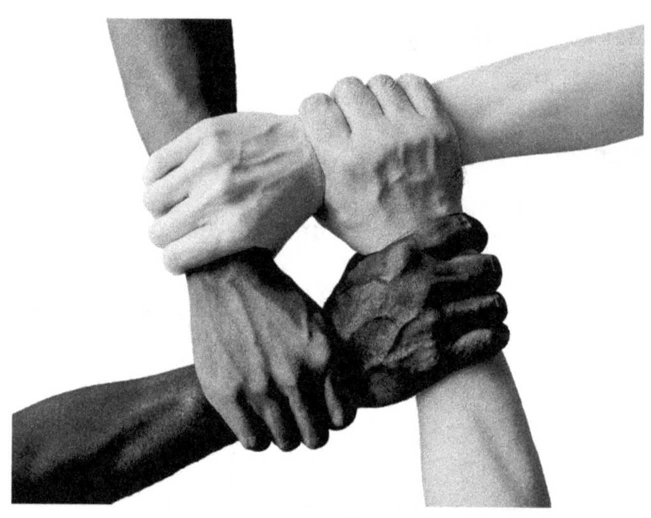

Keep in mind that "birds of a feather do flock together." For this reason, finding a tribe that is positive and uplifting is of utmost importance. Constantly associating with alcoholics, drug addicts, naysayers, negative Nannies, or anyone who puts your dreams down etc., will only drain your life's energy and deplete your opportunities for joy. And believe it or not, staying in the pack will not help your negative friends. Making positive changes will help them see that change is possible. However, if you are in a group of crabs in a bucket pulling each other back into the bucket, realizing your true potential can become a draining seemingly impossible task.

Changing ourselves and being selective about our associates is important not only for ourselves but for the betterment of the world at large. Our communities should uplift us and recharge us, not make us feel depleted and tired. Choose your friends well. As we grow into our true selves, we give others permission to do the same. When the naysayers see your changes, they may also follow you on the path to discover their own journey to find their true selves. And when they do, they may return in love and light to be the true friends you desired, or they may find their own tribe of uplifting people that support and help build their dreams. However, even if the naysayers never change, that is not your fault. All you can do is don the mask of oxygenated yoga breath, peaceful asana practice, mindful meditation, and invigorating chanting on yourself first so that you can then help those you love and others on this rocket ship we call earth.

You may also benefit from finding a yoga community. For over twenty years, my friend's mother Martha, who introduced me to the practice of yoga, looked forward every year to a retreat with her teacher and other students who had become her friends. People who seek to invigorate their lives will also have energy to share. The more people who practice yoga, the better the world will be. When more people are healthy, happy and holy within themselves, they will have no reason to resent, judge, and fear others.

Violence may not disappear, but how society reacts to violence may drastically change. Perhaps society may stop reacting to the whims of a momentarily poisoned child and get the child the antidote it needs to rid itself of the poison. In most cases, a little understanding and kindness would go a long way. And when the poison of resentment and holding grudges festers, it may become the roots of the fairy tale "Evil Queen," who destroys the land and seeks to kill the heroes, namely the rest of humanity. Or worse yet, we may ourselves become the villain in our own and our loved ones' stories when we do not take good care of ourselves. We can see the roots of war and other horrific crimes in the festering of grudges between political leaders with enflamed egos. It is my dream that yoga philosophies of oneness permeate the leaderships of every country of the world, and a true Renaissance emerges out of the ashes of separation that we have left behind, a Renaissance that uplifts every individual by supporting and encouraging all forms of innovations, especially in the realms of living holistically.

On that note, I'd like to specify that yoga is not about homogenizing countries into one, but rather respecting the differences and abundance of all. There are many colors and forms of roses and orchids. And that is how it should be. Encouraging growth and interactions and healing among citizens is not homogenizing but is helping to realize human potential. It is my dream that in countries where women are still treated as slaves and ethnic tribes are treated as pests, when the ruling classes find their humanity, these evils will also cease.

A culture based on the enslavement of other human beings is not a culture we want or need to exist. This is the type of culture that has led to horrific inhumanity, which creates more fear and more war and adds to individual and societal unhappiness. Even those who persecute the innocent live in deplorable fear and inhumanity. These destructive tendencies that may have persisted for most of human existence lead to more and more fear, unworthiness, insecurities, guilt, and general unhealthiness of both individuals and the collective societies in which they live. This disease of the mind, heart, and soul becomes a vicious cycle. Yoga is a powerful tool in disrupting that cycle.

Yoga is a direct path to find our humanity. It is a portal that can take people instantly, even if just for a few moments on the mat, to their true selves. Through the breathing and postures (asanas), we are able to let go and find peace within. And when we go out into the world, we bring that peace with us.

COMPASSION FOR ALL LIVING BEINGS

"He who is cruel to animals becomes hard also in his dealings with men. We can judge the heart of a man by his treatment of animals."– Immanuel Kant

AHIMSA (The art of non-violence)

How we treat ourselves, by allowing others to harm us or engaging in harmful activities, like drugs, too much alcohol, smoking cigarettes etc., is the karma we are creating for ourselves and for this planet. People may not be able to control how others treat them, but they can control how they treat themselves. And unless the person is in a prison or a concentration camp or horrific situation such as this, people can walk away and ask for and accept help, so they can move to living a truly joyous life. I've heard victims of abuse say that they stayed married to an abuser because they thought it was strong to be able to take all the psychological and physical abuse. What these people do not realize is that the more they allow someone to call them stupid and beat them down, the weaker their mind and body becomes. When we realize that by allowing others to harm us, we are not strong, but we are causing harm, not only to ourselves and to those who love us, but to life in general. We may not be able to change an abuser, but we can take ourselves out of harm's way. When we realize the broader effects of our thoughts and actions, being kind to ourselves becomes a very important responsibility.

In our yoga practice and our lives, by observing the body and breath and choosing, to the best of our ability, happy, healthy, holy options with every breath we inhale, with every bite of food or sip of beverage we enjoy, with these precious moments, we are honoring our lives and all living beings.

Anyone who can look into an animal's eyes and not see a soul might want to question, not whether the dog has a soul, but, whether the human in the mirror has one. The answer, whether you believe it or not, is yes. We live such a material existence, that like the cholesterol corroding our arteries, we have gunk coating and hiding our souls. We cannot see in others what we cannot see in ourselves. The practice of yoga, meditation and chanting is to help us clear away the gunk so that our souls can sparkle and shine. And only then will we regain the ability to recognize the precious divinity in all of life.

On that note, if all you see in the mirror of the world is negativity, then you might want to look in the mirror of your soul and take stock of what you see there before blaming the world. We are all microcosms of the macrocosm. As each one of us wakes up, even one, simply by our interactions with each other and with the planet, we are waking up the world's consciousness and in the universe itself. It is logical to say, "Hey, the universe is awake; we don't need to wake it up." And you'd be right. But it is not awake in us, and that is the most important part for our human evolution on this planet.

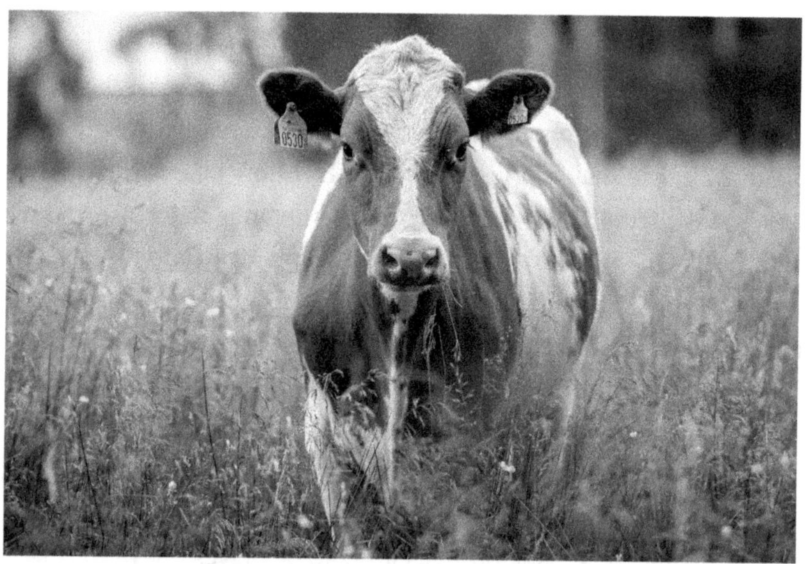

We are the guardians, the caretakers; we are not the great destroyers. Destruction may appear to be the human manifesto, but it is not our mission. And for those who have risen to their true calling, an inner peace and happiness is the result of such courage. It does take courage to be the lotus flower in the mud. It takes courage to stand-up to injustice when we encounter it. It takes courage to live with morals and principals that include compassion for all living beings, including humans that may appear as enemies. It takes courage to look within oneself and feel someone else's pain, to empathize rather than sit afar, unaffected, expressing meaningless sympathies rather than demonstrating true compassion.

The next logical step from empathy is action. It was first empathy that prompted the great movements of change, not empathy only for others, but also for oneself. To truly feel how we would feel, in a similar situation as another, is the beginning of truly feeling the pain, we have often created in our own lives that we numb with food, alcohol, drugs, television, and any other over-indulgent activity.

Through the action of the practice of yoga and meditation we are brought back to the body and the breath and the present moment, which we are standing in right now, time and time again. Yoga asks nothing other than to be present with where you are in this precious moment, to allow the tears to flow if they choose to, to allow pain to be felt and released through the breath, to allow the body and mind to heal and be rejuvenated, to repair the old hurts and wounds that the body and muscles may be holding so that the mind does not have to hold them, which causes toxins and pain in the muscles. The body is not really a collection of separate parts but is, instead, a vessel for a whole being. Yoga is a holistic practice, and with compassion for ourselves on the mat, we can develop even more compassion for others in the world.

Evolution of the Soul

Sometimes we may feel like we are dying when we release old ideas. However, we die a little throughout our lives as we grow from a baby to become a toddler then a young child and later an adolescent and a young adult then a mature adult and so on. Each time we gradually change in often dramatic ways, even though this change is imperceptible in the moment, it is happening before our eyes. In the same way, the world is witnessing a remarkable transformation. The benefits and transformative powers of yoga, if practiced daily for a lifetime are multiplied as the world transforms with us. As we transform, we encourage others by our actions to do the same. And as others transform to live as their true selves, we are bolstered to continue growing. In so doing, we are creating a healing cycle for all human life, and ultimately, all life on the planet will benefit from this human transformation.

There are many religions of the world that view death and rebirth as a fact of life. Buddhism is one. The Buddha, Siddhartha Gautama discovered birth, death, sickness and suffering and longed to find meaning and to help others find happiness amidst these harsh realities of life. And many Christians believe that the suffering, death, and resurrection of Jesus are also symbols for our own power of transformation. At first spiritual, physical and mental transformation may seem daunting, but after a resurrection when we have been transported to the other side of our problems, we may have moments of peace as never before. Of course, we eventually see this as normal and continue to strive to move our souls and current lives further in the direction of the realm of true happiness. However, as we move our lives in the direction of true humanity, we often discover more obstacles to help us continue to transform and grow as bodhisattvas of the Earth.

A good explanation of a bodhisattvas is a person who is on the path of achieving enlightenment in this lifetime, in other words a Buddha, one who experiences eternity, happiness, true self, and purity and refers to the supreme state we can attain as human beings, a state of absolute freedom and happiness. And in Nicheren Buddhism / SGI, Soka Gaki International, which means value creating society, a bodhisattva is also someone who leads others to this true state of pure happiness, a state that is not altered by the winds of external circumstances.

In yoga, obstacles may come in the form of time, other commitments, our bodies changing, even an instructor. In these moments and times, we must honor our bodies and listen to its needs, honor the needs of those we love and our commitments such as jobs etc., but we must also honor our growth and inherent need and right to health, balance and compassion. These are gifts we must give ourselves each day. They were given to most of us at birth; it is our job to maintain the working order of these gifts with respect and love for ourselves and others.

Still there are other obstacles that manifest in even more powerful forms. There are many terminal and destructive illnesses plaguing our society today like the big ones, cancer, heart disease, and diabetes; and increasing ones, dementia, Alzheimer's, ALS, Amyotrophic lateral sclerosis. Is it possible that as a species on this earth, our collective karma is affecting all of life on the planet including individual human lives?

The word sickness in the four universal sufferings of birth, aging, sickness, and death, may be misunderstood to mean that sickness is inevitable. Death is inevitable. Sickness is a state of being. However, even if we die peacefully in our sleep, we will have experienced some form of physical illness even if it was a simple common cold or an innocuous accidental food poisoning. And we will all age, which has its own set of sufferings, from physical restrictions to psychological consequences.

The goal of this book is to help humans live as our vibrant selves while we are alive. Our bodies were designed to expire so that we may move on in our growth and transformation through the cycles of birth, aging, sickness, and death. But while we are here, it is our job to do everything in our power to assist in this growth, to water and feed our souls and bodies nutrition that is loving and compassionate, substances and experiences that not only help to heal our suffering, but the suffering of the world. In Buddhism as more and more individuals become enlightened to the reality of life and achieving true happiness, not the fleeting happiness of life circumstances, then we as a species may make that quantum leap to enlightenment for all. In Buddhism, each person's practice for themselves and others is that important.

CHANTING

THE BASICS OF BUDDHISM

I was fortunate last month to have the opportunity to deeply ponder the question of Buddhism when my local chapter asked me to give a lecture at a group meeting explaining the basics of the practice.

WHAT IS BUDDHISM?

There are libraries full of books on Buddhism that I encourage you to explore. This book again is designed to give those who had no knowledge of yoga a sample of the practice and a taste of Buddhism so that they might go on their own journeys to discover the infinite world that lives within each of us.

For a quick definition, Buddhism began roughly twenty-five hundred years ago. Shakyamuni Buddha, also known as Siddhartha Gautama, abandoned his life as a prince in India to seek a means to end human suffering. His teachings culminated in the Lotus Sutra, which elucidates the eternally present Buddha nature inherent in all life.

WHAT IS NICHIREN BUDDHISM?

Nichiren Daishonin, a reformer in thirteenth century Japan, studied the writings of Buddhism for many years and realized that the Lotus Sutra was the supreme teaching. The title of this sutra translates from its original Sanskrit to ancient Chinese as "Myoho Renge Kyo." Nam was added to the beginning of this chant, which in Sanskrit means, "devotion to." Along with two chapters of the Lotus Sutra, this is the chant that practitioners of Nicheren Buddhism typically recite.

WHY DO WE CHANT?

Nichiren realized that chanting, "Nam Myoho Renge Kyo," made Buddhism available to all people, as the original Buddha intended. While Siddhartha's previous writings that say enlightenment will take many lifetimes or kalpas are considered provisionary teachings in order to prepare the people of that time for the truth, the Lotus Sutra states that we can attain enlightenment or Buddhahood in this lifetime.

HOW CAN THIS BE?

The words "Nam Myoho Renge Kyo," are also ancient Sanskrit seed sounds, which are believed to be thousands of years old, perhaps even predating known civilizations. I recently saw a NASA youtube.com video of the sounds recorded from the sun and our solar system. Scientists were amazed to discover that the universe makes sounds. Scientists have also discovered that sounds are also vibrations and that everything in existence is made up of energy vibrating at various frequencies. By chanting, we connect to the Mystic Law of the universe, also called the unfathomable that permeates all existence.

There have been many paths that people have walked to become one with universal truths. People have asked me, "What is the difference between meditation and chanting?" I have been an avid practitioner of meditation for over thirty years. It has great benefits to relieve stress and calm the psyche and even relieve muscle tension and assist in healing the mind, body and soul as I have reviewed in the yoga weeks of this book. I have had great insights both sitting in quiet meditation listening to the voice that is within me, and in vibrantly and powerfully chanting Nam Myoho Renge Kyo.

However, action is what changes our karma. Several Buddhism books liken chanting to "when a caged bird sings." Our karma and minds have caged us, but when we sing (chant), we begin to shatter the illusion of the cage that holds us and begin to realize our true boundless potential. Chanting is the engine and the fuel that transforms karma. Being a direct connection to the mystic law, universal consciousness, I liken chanting to taking the TGV, the fast train in France to wherever I want to go. Meditation is a similar but different tool to awakening our true-selves and to transforming both our own and our collective human karma.

Unlike the revelations from quiet meditation, the engine of chanting has given me the courage to take action, to do things previously unimaginable and to overcome fear and doubts. It dispels the fears and fuels my determination to transform my karma in this lifetime and to transform my life to living joyfully each moment of each day. During one of my first experiences with chanting, tears flowed down my face as heartfelt love flowed, and I was able to forgive someone who greatly harmed me. I may not always be able to laugh at obstacles, but at least I have the determination to overcome them and the knowledge that I can. With the power, knowledge, and wisdom of this practice, I am unstoppable in achieving my goals and taking steps forward, not only for my own benefit but for the benefit of all living beings.

Chanting for the benefit of others is a basic component of the practice of Nicheren Buddhism. I have always wanted to help others in any way that I was able. It took me many years to realize that the best way I could help others was to show them the power of my own transformation, to be the change I wished to see in the world. When people see our joy and feel the energy of our happiness and our resolve to overcome every obstacle in the path of our goals and our enlightenment, they will be inspired to learn more and hopefully desire to thrive in a similar way.

One very special time, I realized the universal truth of transforming ourselves first was at a yoga teacher training. I noticed that Eliza, a fellow yoga student was struggling. She had stomach problems and seemed very unhappy. She could not rid herself of parasites in her gut that had been plaguing her for several years. These parasites seemed to not just be living in her gut and off her life force, but also consuming her joy. Another student, Rebecca, noticed my frustration with Eliza, who would rebuff my suggestions, saying that she had tried everything. I had been struggling in trying to advise Eliza on her diet and that medical doctors, although well-meaning, since after years had not found a solution, may not know a solution. I was genuinely trying to help her. Rebecca encouraged me to just be myself and to let go of trying to convince or change others. I finally took this advice, and on the last day of our classes, Eliza approached me with tears in her eyes and said that I reminded her of how she used to be, that my happiness and playfulness was how she used to be before she was ill. She genuinely thanked me for existing and being myself. I really wanted to connect with Eliza and to help her, and when I realized that being an living example was enough, I was overjoyed with tearful delight as well. Perhaps my life condition was the memory of hope she needed to transform the parasitic obstacles that had been plaguing her life.

WHAT IS THE SGI?

SGI stands for Soka Gakkai International and translates to "Value Creating Society." It is the lay Buddhist organization, practicing and promoting world peace through Nicheren Buddhism. The organization's last president, Daisaku Ikeda said, "A great human revolution in just a single individual will help achieve a change in the destiny of a nation and further, will enable a change in the destiny of all humankind." The SGI is an organization of practitioners in 192 countries who not only chant together, but by being living examples of the power to transform their karma and their lives, they give each other boundless encouragement and hope.

There are many other aspects to Nichiren Buddhism such as a Gohonzon, the mandala that represents the mirror of the soul, and Gongyo, the practice of chanting in the morning and evening. I encourage anyone inspired to transform their lives to overcome all obstacles by living as their true selves, and interested in the great benefit of supporting others and being supported by other positive, empowered people, to go to the site listed below for more detailed information and to find a chapter near you.

http://www.sgi.org (International)

http://www.sgi-usa.org

https://buddhability.org

SKIN-DEEP

Beauty is not skin-deep. Beauty emerges from the inside out. I had a friend in college who was constantly making angry faces. I warned her that if she didn't stop doing that, her pretty face would soon become mean and ugly. I was watching this process happen before my eyes. I did not see her for years, but thankfully, she learned to curb her propensity to make mean faces. When I saw her last, she was smiling for no real reason. It was a pleasure to see that she did not ruin her face but was more beautiful twenty years later than she had ever been in her twenties. We could say that smiling and a joyful attitude are worth their weight in expensive face creams.

How do facial expressions affect us in deeper, more meaningful ways? An actor knows that contorting his face into an angry grimace can help him evoke the feeling of anger to pull from the gut for an intended response. I used this technique to emote the correct emotions for tears to flow every night for the opening scene in the play, House of Bernarda Alba. I began my rehearsals by listening to a sad song, which also worked for performances. Music is also a catalyst for our emotional state. With practice however, I stopped needing the music. I would force my facial muscles into sadness, and the tears would begin to flow naturally.

We can make ourselves happy, sad, angry or relaxed in many ways by our own intentions. When we walk around with a heavy heart or anger, or with slumped, defeated shoulders, we are also projecting this image out into the world. We not only tell others who we are in that moment by our facial expressions and body language, more importantly, we tell ourselves, and we get the message loud and clear.

I had a friend who explained that he had anger issues and that this is just who he is and who he had always been. Even though I explained that he could change this very unhealthy state of being with chanting, meditation, and yoga, he did not believe me. If you think you are angry, smart, beautiful, kind, mean, dumb, etc. that is what you will be. That is the power of the mind and the power of programming. Changing childhood programming, as in my friend's case, may seem impossible, but it is not.

The practice of yoga, meditation, and chanting are about accepting ourselves where we are and then developing the courage and the strength to change. Change, like death, is a reality of life. When we stop changing and growing, the alternative is that we begin dying rather than vibrantly living.

WE ARE ALL STARS

"We are all playing a leading role, having taken our place in this trouble-filled *saha* world to act out the drama of kosen rufu."

❋ Daisaku Ikeda, The Wisdom of the Lotus Sutra, Volume 1, p. 129.

After reading this passage, I asked myself, "how do humans choose their characters?" I saw how each of us is playing the part of our own drama, our play. In Buddhism it is believed that we have chosen our current existence with all of its obstacles and mishaps. We have chosen to live in this world to transform and help others to transform. And in Buddhist and yoga traditions, evolution and transformation are our ultimate purpose.

Still, I have heard several friends tell me that they cannot control their thoughts. The idea that we are not our thoughts seemed very foreign to them. I began to wonder if symptoms of mental illness are the cause of their random, negative thoughts or if years of the perpetuation of negative, self-defeating thoughts are the cause of mental illness. Is it possible that the brain's wiring and ability to produce the appropriate or healthy chemical reactions could be affected by repeated and perpetual negative thinking? I asked this because we are living in an age where mental illness seems an epidemic. More and more children are put on mind and physical altering drugs to control their outbursts and behaviors. More and more adults are succumbing to depression and other related illnesses like bi-polar disorder, which appears to need life-long medical treatment.

And there are other forms of epidemic mental illnesses, for instance, the ability to choose to murder hundreds of thousands of people rather than to choose a place of peace to have rational conversations. The strike first, talk second, murder doesn't matter if it's called war mentality is also an epidemic in our current and historical societies. Unfortunately, this epidemic or drama has been going on since the dawn of Earth and human time. People have suffered from the insane illusion that killing is okay if it is a means to an end. Unfortunately, so many returning soldiers are also diagnosed with PTS disorders and are prescribed medications to deal with the stress of returning home to an environment where every noise in the night is likely not a bomb going off. What is the drama or play that we as a collective are creating that puts young women and men in harms-way to prove a point or to make more money for the very wealthy or to secure "our" interests in regions we do not belong in anyway? How can we as a collective change this fear-based drama that dooms us to repeated misery?

I think starting with the dramas we create in our own homes and heads might be a very good place to start. I am not a psychiatrist, nor a doctor of any kind. I am merely a person who questions and observes. I question whether drugs, which have so many side effects, can ultimately solve people's problems. I wonder if taking spoonfuls of happy thoughts, through chanting, yoga, meditation, and exercise is a better way to cure the blues. I have known people who seemed completely unable to perceive anything positive. A friend, Cindy told our mutual friend, Amy, "I will never get married, and no one will ever love me." Amy told Cindy, "With that attitude, you will never be married or loved." How are we manifesting exactly what we think will happen? How do we change from manifesting our worst fears to living our most beautiful dreams?

I may not be a doctor, but I am an actor and have transformed inside and out on stage and on camera to manifest the emotions and the moments the scenes needed to tell the story the directors envisioned. Perhaps we are all the directors, the actors and the writers for the scenes of our lives. I am also a screenwriter and have used the skill of visualizing how I'd like a scene to go, not only on the page but also in my "real" life. Once, I was afraid of the potential anger my friend might have when I asked her to move out of my apartment. I saw the anger very clearly. I chanted, "Nam Myoho Renge Kyo" to clear my mind of negative, fearful thoughts. While chanting, I began to feel better. I then began visualizing the outcome I desired, a calm, rational, sincere conversation. I began to feel more and more certain that there would be a positive outcome to our discussion. I was relieved and filled with gratitude when this vision of peace is what I manifested that day.

If I had entered that conversation with the fear and resentment that I previously felt, my fears would have manifested. I knew I had to speak from a place of love and respect, and that this place had to be created by me. The friend I had to have this conversation with also suffers from a mental illness, so I had that fear to deal with as well. But I was able to overcome not only my own fundamental darkness that day, but possibly her fundamental darkness as well. And that is the tip of the iceberg of the power of adding chanting to your daily yoga practice.

How can we, as individual cities, states, countries, and continents come together with our collective dysfunctional characters to instead choose peaceful roles, leaving the fundamental darkness at the door? If the political figures we choose to elect could come to the table of dialogue from a place of truth and compassion and ultimately true power rather than fear, we may begin to see the end of one form of collective mental illness, war. And aren't the atrocities that plague the world in the form of genocide, human female mutilation, mass killings and beheadings, all the atrocities that happen in the world, even treating animals like machines and torturing and killing eight billion of these innocent creatures in the United States alone, aren't these all symptoms of mass mental illness? To quote a dear friend, "The inmates are running the asylum." The people of the world have allowed people suffering with severe mental illnesses to be the leaders of society for far too long. Isn't it time we put stock in commodities that have a chance to yield the positive, empowered, abundant results we desire?

I realized when dealing with my own drama about asking my friend to move, I had to change the character I was choosing to play, from one of stress and fear and resignation to one empowered with truth and emblazoned with the light of compassion. During rehearsals, actors are constantly refining their characters, questioning their motives and the inner obstacles to that character's success. Perhaps these same skills can be used to refine and fine-tune our own characters in the world as well. If the world is all a stage, then let us play our best characters in this amazing production. Let us overcome every obstacle to our enlightenment with courage and compassion. Let us lift our hearts and our hands to help others and thereby help ourselves, for as the energy of each individual transforms and is raised to a higher consciousness, so too is the consciousness of all of creation.

The yoga lessons and complementary practices listed in this book have worked for me to overcome many obstacles and to live my life with more youthful vigor. I know that the path of yoga and working towards enlightenment may not be for everyone, but for those reading this book, it is. We are all individuals in a giant field of energy, sharing our energy with everyone we encounter and even those we do not know. Yoga, meditation, and chanting are tools to keep us centered in an often-chaotic world. We do not have the power to control other people's responses or even the circumstances of the world as a whole; however, we do have the power to control our thoughts and whether we choose to react impulsively or to resist this temptation and choose our truth and peaceful wisdom instead. When we emerge from the land of peace within ourselves after our yoga, meditation, and chanting-for-world-peace practice, creating a peaceful existence becomes a reality. To infuse peace in our actions, we must first have peace within ourselves. Our health, well-being, and interactions are our responsibilities and gifts, not only, to ourselves, but also to the immediate world we live in and the collective universal world of pure consciousness. By dipping into the ocean of peace through practicing yoga, we are filling our minds, bodies, and souls with inner peace every day.

A FEW FAVORITES

Yoga

Light On Yoga by BKS Iyengar

Light on Pranayama by BKS Iyengar

Light on Life by BKS Iyengar

The Five Tibetans by Christopher S. Kilham

Autobiography of a Yogi by Paramahasa Yogananda

Kundalini Yoga by Shakti Parwha Kaur Khalsa

Kriya: Yoga Sets, Meditations, & Classic Kriyas by Yogi Bhajan

Ashtanga Yoga: The Practice Manual by David Swenson

Enlightenment and Buddhism

The Buddha in the Mirror Woody Hochswender, Greg Martin & Ted Mornino

The Wisdom of the Lotus Sutra by Daisaku Ikeda

The Miracle of Mindfulness: An Introduction to the Practice of Meditation by Thich Nhat Hanh

The Power of Now: A Guide to Spiritual Enlightenment by Eckhart Tolle

A New Earth: Awakening to Your Life's Purpose by Eckhart Tolle

Unlocking the Mysteries of Birth & Death…And Everything in Between, A Buddhist View of Life by Daisaku Ikeda

Syncrodestiny by Deepak Chopra

Happiness Becomes You by Tina Turner

Wherever You Go, There You Are by Jon Kabat-Zinn

You Can Heal Your Life by Louise Hay

The Life Changing Magic of Tidying Up by Marie Kondo

Diet

Diet for a New America by John Robbins

The Gerson Therapy by Charlotte Gerson and Morton Walker D.P.M.

Master Cleanser by Stanley Burroughs

Green For Life, Victoria Boutenko

Rainbow Green Live-Food Cuisine by Gabriel Cousens, MD

What the Health film by Kip Anderson and Keegan Kuhn

Seaspiracy film by Ali Tabrizi and Kip and Anderson

Music

Sean Johnson and the Wild Lotus Band

Nirinjan Kaur

Krisna Das